For Dummies™
BESTSELLING BOOK SERIES

P9-DOA-184

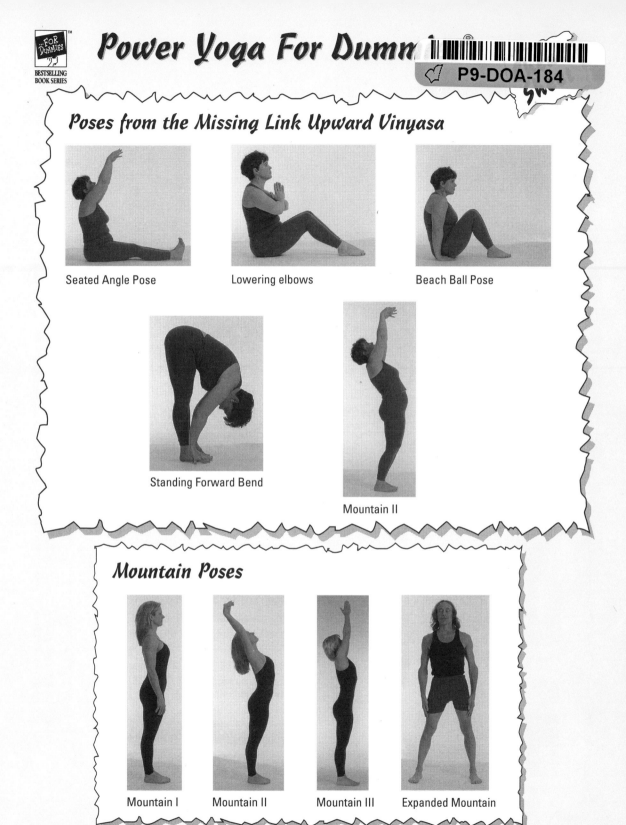

Poses from the Missing Link Upward Vinyasa

Seated Angle Pose

Lowering elbows

Beach Ball Pose

Standing Forward Bend

Mountain II

Mountain Poses

Mountain I

Mountain II

Mountain III

Expanded Mountain

For Dummies: Bestselling Book Series for Beginners

Power Yoga For Dummies®

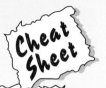
Cheat Sheet

Common Power Yoga Poses

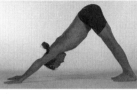

Downward Facing Dog

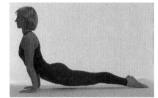

Upward Facing Dog

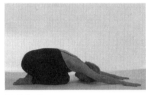

Child's Pose

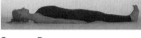

Corpse Pose

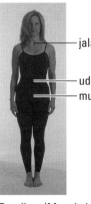

— jalandhara bandha

— uddiyana bandha
— mula bandha

Bandhas (Muscle locks)

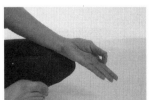

Jnana Mudra

Yoga Breathing

Incorporate proper Yoga breathing, called *ujjayi*, in every Power Yoga pose. You know you have it down when you make a slight purring or hissing sound as you inhale and exhale.

1. **Sit comfortably.**
2. **Close your eyes and inhale slowly through your nose, fully expanding your lungs.**
3. **Exhale just as slowly through your nose.**
4. **Keep breathing through your nose and tighten your throat muscles a bit as you whisper "haaaaa" through your mouth.**
5. **Continue breathing deeply and slowly, feeling and hearing the air passing through your slightly tightened throat and over the roof of your mouth.**

Copyright © 2001 Wiley Publishing, Inc. All rights reserved.

Cheat Sheet $2.95 value. Item 5342-9.

For more information about Wiley Publishing, call 1-800-762-2974.

Wiley, the Wiley Publishing logo, For Dummies, the Dummies Man logo, the For Dummies Bestselling Book Series logo and all related trade dress are trademarks or registered trademarks of Wiley Publishing, Inc. All other trademarks are property of their respective owners.

For Dummies: Bestselling Book Series for Beginners

Praise for Power Yoga For Dummies

"*Power Yoga For Dummies* is a lot of fun to read! It is an excellent reference book with plenty of snippets of handy information. Flipping through the pages is an easy way to ferret out some of the Yoga fundamentals without making a pilgrimage to India. You can open this book to any page, at any point, on any day, and receive some inspirational guidance that would be a benefit to your life at that moment."

> — Beryl Bender Birch, director, The Hard & Soft Astanga Yoga Institute, author of *Beyond Power Yoga*

"In *Power Yoga For Dummies*, Doug Swenson masterfully presents one of the most physically challenging styles of hathaYoga in a way students of any level will find safe, fun, easeful, and empowering. Doug Swenson's creative postural modifications and variations of some of the standard Power Yoga poses and sequences will surely influence the evolution of the modern practice of hathaYoga throughout the world."

> — John Friend, founder of AnusaraYoga

"Doug Swenson is a real Yogi, one in a million. He is living it and doing it 100%. We are fortunate that Doug has taken the time to share his knowledge and experience of Yoga, a subject that we all find so fascinating. My best wishes go to Doug in this endeavor and to all who are fortunate enough to have this book and Yoga come into their lives."

> — David Williams, daily practitioner of Yoga since 1971

"Doug Swenson has created a book about Yoga that captures his delightful and unique teaching style. This is not only an excellent practice manual, it is also a wonderful, humor-filled journey into the practice of power Yoga for both the beginner and more experienced student, in which he anticipates and addresses the many questions that arise along the way."

> — Karen Allen, actress, practicing Yogini

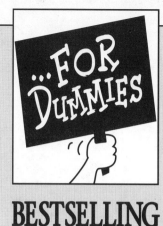

TM

References for the Rest of Us!®

BESTSELLING BOOK SERIES

Do you find that traditional reference books are overloaded with technical details and advice you'll never use? Do you postpone important life decisions because you just don't want to deal with them? Then our *For Dummies*® business and general reference book series is for you.

For Dummies business and general reference books are written for those frustrated and hard-working souls who know they aren't dumb, but find that the myriad of personal and business issues and the accompanying horror stories make them feel helpless. *For Dummies* books use a lighthearted approach, a down-to-earth style, and even cartoons and humorous icons to dispel fears and build confidence. Lighthearted but not lightweight, these books are perfect survival guides to solve your everyday personal and business problems.

"More than a publishing phenomenon, 'Dummies' is a sign of the times."

— The New York Times

"A world of detailed and authoritative information is packed into them..."

— U.S. News and World Report

"...you won't go wrong buying them."

— Walter Mossberg, Wall Street Journal, on For Dummies books

Already, millions of satisfied readers agree. They have made For Dummies the #1 introductory level computer book series and a best-selling business book series. They have written asking for more. So, if you're looking for the best and easiest way to learn about business and other general reference topics, look to For Dummies to give you a helping hand.

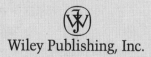

Wiley Publishing, Inc.

5/09

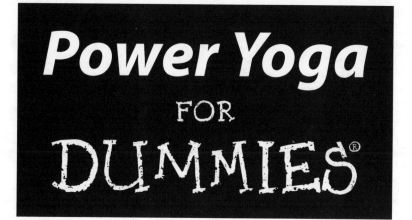

by Doug Swenson

Foreword by David Swenson

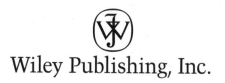

Wiley Publishing, Inc.

Power Yoga For Dummies®

Published by
Wiley Publishing, Inc.
909 Third Avenue
New York, NY 10022
www.wiley.com

Copyright © 2001 by Wiley Publishing, Inc., Indianapolis, Indiana

Published simultaneously in Canada

No part of this publication may be reproduced, stored in a retrieval system, or transmitted in any form or by any means, electronic, mechanical, photocopying, recording, scanning, or otherwise, except as permitted under Sections 107 or 108 of the 1976 United States Copyright Act, without either the prior written permission of the Publisher, or authorization through payment of the appropriate per-copy fee to the Copyright Clearance Center, 222 Rosewood Drive, Danvers, MA 01923, 978-750-8400, fax 978-750-4744. Requests to the Publisher for permission should be addressed to the Legal Department, Wiley Publishing, Inc., 10475 Crosspoint Blvd., Indianapolis, IN 46256, 317-572-3447, fax 317-572-4447, or e-mail permcoordinator@wiley.com

Trademarks: Wiley, the Wiley Publishing logo, For Dummies, the Dummies Man logo, A Reference for the Rest of Us!, The Dummies Way, Dummies Daily, The Fun and Easy way, Dummies.com and related trade dress are trademarks or registered trademarks of Wiley Publishing, Inc., in the United States and other countries, and may not be used without written permission. All other trademarks are the property of their respective owners. Wiley Publishing, Inc., is not associated with any product or vendor mentioned in this book.

LIMIT OF LIABILITY/DISCLAIMER OF WARRANTY: WHILE THE PUBLISHER AND AUTHOR HAVE USED THEIR BEST EFFORTS IN PREPARING THIS BOOK, THEY MAKE NO REPRESENTATIONS OR WARRANTIES WITH RESPECT TO THE ACCURACY OR COMPLETENESS OF THE CONTENTS OF THIS BOOK AND SPECIFICALLY DISCLAIM ANY IMPLIED WARRANTIES OF MERCHANTABILITY OR FITNESS FOR A PARTICULAR PURPOSE. NO WARRANTY MAY BE CREATED OR EXTENDED BY SALES REPRESENTATIVES OR WRITTEN SALES MATERIALS. THE ADVICE AND STRATEGIES CONTAINED HEREIN MAY NOT BE SUITABLE FOR YOUR SITUATION. YOU SHOULD CONSULT WITH A PROFESSIONAL WHERE APPROPRIATE. NEITHER THE PUBLISHER NOR AUTHOR SHALL BE LIABLE FOR ANY LOSS OF PROFIT OR ANY OTHER COMMERCIAL DAMAGES, INCLUDING BUT NOT LIMITED TO SPECIAL, INCIDENTAL, CONSEQUENTIAL, OR OTHER DAMAGES. THE INFORMATION IN THIS REFERENCE IS NOT INTENDED TO SUBSTITUTE FOR EXPERT MEDICAL ADVICE OR TREATMENT; IT IS DESIGNED TO HELP YOU MAKE INFORMED CHOICES. BECAUSE EACH INDIVIDUAL IS UNIQUE, A PHYSICIAN OR OTHER QUALIFIED HEALTH CARE PRACTITIONER MUST DIAGNOSE CONDITIONS AND SUPERVISE TREATMENTS FOR EACH INDIVIDUAL HEALTH PROBLEM. IF AN INDIVIDUAL IS UNDER A DOCTOR OR OTHER QUALIFIED HEALTH CARE PRACTITIONER'S CARE AND RECEIVES ADVICE CONTRARY TO INFORMATION PROVIDED IN THIS REFERENCE, THE DOCTOR OR OTHER QUALIFIED HEALTH CARE PRACTITIONER'S ADVICE SHOULD BE FOLLOWED, AS IT IS BASED ON THE UNIQUE CHARACTERISTICS OF THAT INDIVIDUAL.

For general information on our other products and services or to obtain technical support, please contact our Customer Care Department within the U.S. at 800-762-2974, outside the U.S. at 317-572-3993, or fax 317-572-4002.

Wiley also publishes its books in a variety of electronic formats. Some content that appears in print may not be available in electronic books.

Library of Congress Cataloging-in-Publication Data:

Library of Congress Control Number: 00-112137
ISBN: 0-7645-5342-9

Manufactured in the United States of America
10 9 8 7 6 5 4 3
1O/RW/QY/QS/IN

About the Author

Doug Swenson is an internationally known Yoga teacher and health educator. Doug began studying Yoga in 1969 with Dr. Ernest Wood and has been practicing and teaching Yoga ever since. Doug has studied under many great teachers, including K. Pattabhi Jois, guru of Ashtanga Yoga, from which Power Yoga was born. Doug has dedicated his life to a holistic approach of Yoga, learning from several different systems, and combining them with his interest in nutrition, concern for the environment, and warm, humorous approach to life to create his own unique and powerful system of Yoga practice. Doug teaches Yoga workshops and teacher-training courses across the U.S. and in other countries. Doug is the author of three books on Yoga, and another on diet and nutrition. Check him out in Chapter 15, doing the Moonbeam Bird in Figure 15-2.

Author's Acknowledgments

Writing a book is a long and often very difficult process. I would have never been able to tackle this project on my own, so I'd like to give my thanks and appreciation to all those who have worked so hard and with such creative energy to help me see it through.

I first want to thank Karen Young (Acquisitions Editor), who is not only a wonderful worker, but also a really cool woman, and who helped me from the very beginning. I'd also like to thank Stacy Klein (Acquisitions Coordinator), Tracy Boggier (Acquisitions Manager), Lee Edgren (Technical Reviewer), Raul Marroquin (Photographer), and Gwenette Gaddis (Copy Editor) for their excellent work. Lorna Gentry (Professional Writing Assistant) polished my work and made it into a wonderful book. Kathleen Dobie (Project Editor) has encouraged and inspired me with suggestions and moral support when the work ahead seemed overwhelming. Carol Susan Roth (Literary Agent) brought me to this wonderful publisher and helped me see the project through.

Additional thanks: I would also like to thank my brother, Master Ashtanga teacher David Swenson, for his support and encouragement and for writing the foreword to this book. I also would like to thank Beryl Bender, author of *Power Yoga* and *Beyond Power Yoga*, for taking the time out of her busy life to write a blurb for this book. If it weren't for the teachings and work of David Williams and Nancy Gilgoff (two of the first and best American teachers of Ashtanga Yoga) this information would not be available today. I would also like to thank the talented actress Karen Allen for her kind words and wonderful friendship. I would like to give special thanks to John Friend for taking time and energy out of his busy schedule to acknowledge this work. John has truly influenced endless Yoga students with his wonderful style of teaching Yoga.

Photo models: I would like to give special thanks to my good friends and photo models: Robert Boustany — Good friend and great yoga teacher, inventor, and philosopher; Anne — Good friend, great yogini, and rock climber; Lisa Wheeler — Friend and kind, sweet yogini; Raye Lynne Rath — Good friend and great Yoga teacher; David Swenson (Brother) — Master Ashtanga teacher and blood brother; Julie Wilkinson — Wonderful yogini and teaching assistant, very close personal friend; Violet Swenson (Mother) — My mother, yogini, and really kindhearted woman. My thanks to a good friend and Yogini model Susan Baker, who has provided wonderful Yoga classes in Northwest Houston for many years.

Publisher's Acknowledgments

We're proud of this book; please send us your comments through our online registration form located at www.dummies.com/register.

Some of the people who helped bring this book to market include the following:

Acquisitions, Editorial, and Media Development

Project Editor: Kathleen A. Dobie

Acquisitions Editor: Karen Young

Copy Editor: Gwenette Gaddis

Acquisitions Coordinator: Stacy Klein

Technical Editor: Lee Edgren

Editorial Manager: Christine Meloy Beck

Editorial Assistants: Jennifer Young, Melissa Bennett

Cover Photo: © Michael Newman Photo Edit/PictureQuest

Interior Photos: Raul Marroquin

Production

Project Coordinator: Nancee Reeves

Layout and Graphics: Jackie Nicholas, Brent Savage, Jacque Schneider, Julie Trippetti, Kristin Pickett

Proofreaders: Nancy Price, Marianne Santy, TECHBOOKS Production Services

Indexer: TECHBOOKS Production Services

Special Help Tere Drenth

Publishing and Editorial for Consumer Dummies
> **Diane Graves Steele,** Vice President and Publisher, Consumer Dummies
> **Joyce Pepple,** Acquisitions Director, Consumer Dummies
> **Kristin A. Cocks,** Product Development Director, Consumer Dummies
> **Michael Spring,** Vice President and Publisher, Travel
> **Brice Gosnell,** Publishing Director, Travel
> **Suzanne Jannetta,** Editorial Director, Travel

Publishing for Technology Dummies
> **Richard Swadley,** Vice President and Executive Group Publisher
> **Andy Cummings,** Vice President and Publisher

Composition Services
> **Gerry Fahey,** Vice President of Production Services
> **Debbie Stailey,** Director of Composition Services

Contents at a Glance

Cartoons at a Glance

By Rich Tennant

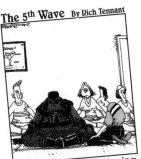

"Okay, you've got the breathing down, but wouldn't you be more comfortable in a different workout suit?"

page 37

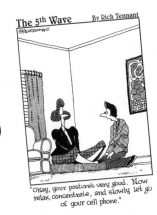

"Okay, your posture's very good. Now relax, concentrate, and slowly let go of your cell phone."

page 7

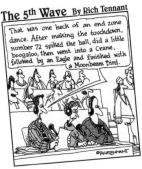

That was one heck of an end zone dance. After making the touchdown, number 72 spiked the ball, did a little boogaloo, then went into a Crane, followed by an Eagle and finished with a Moonbeam Bird.

page 313

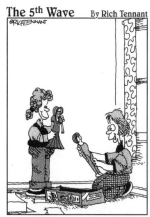

"...and this one's Yogini Barbie. She doesn't come with a lot of stuff, but you can bend her into 13 different positions without anything breaking."

page 225

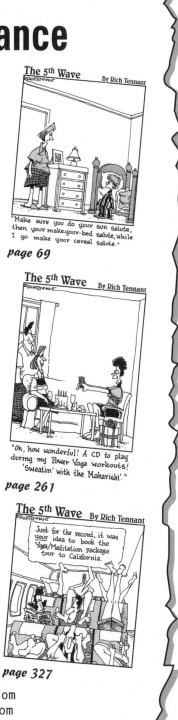

"Make sure you do your sun salute, then your make-your-bed salute, while I go make your cereal salute."

page 69

"Oh, how wonderful! A CD to play during my Power Yoga workouts! 'Sweatin' with the Maharishi'."

page 261

Just for the record, it was your idea to book the Yoga/Meditation package tour to California.

page 327

Cartoon Information:
Fax: 978-546-7747
E-Mail: richtennant@the5thwave.com
World Wide Web: www.the5thwave.com

Table of Contents

Foreword

T here was a time when the words "power" and "yoga" would have been considered out of place in the same sentence. In the past, yoga was thought of as being graceful, but few would have considered it to be powerful as well. But I think that we too often fail to recognize the many ways that grace and power go hand in hand, particularly in nature. A gently flowing stream, a flower stretching toward the sun, and a bird gliding upon the wind all demonstrate quite graceful yet powerful acts of nature. The same close marriage of grace and power shines through in the practice of Power Yoga.

Doug Swenson is not only my biological brother but he is also the one who introduced me to the magical world of yoga, and its integral ties to good health and natural living. Doug teaches by example; he has been a dedicated practitioner of yoga for three decades. In 1977 he authored one of America's first yoga books: *Yoga Helps*. Though Doug is well-known for his humorous and openhearted approach to teaching, he is a serious yogi who "walks his talk" in every way. In writing *Power Yoga For Dummies*, Doug has once again demonstrated his skills as an instructor by presenting a complex body of knowledge in a down-to-earth format. Doug's book offers a well-rounded look at this popular form of yoga — from its early roots to its present-day expression. *Power Yoga For Dummies* is a perfect introduction to Yoga for any newcomer and it will be a welcome addition to the bookshelves of seasoned Yoga practitioners.

David Swenson

Introduction

*I*t seems that just yesterday, Yoga was practiced only by incredibly enlight-ened people in the Far East — very few people in the Western world even knew about Yoga. You may not have even considered looking at a book on Yoga until recently, and now here you are with a Power Yoga book in your hands.

Well, time passes, as it always seems to do! In just a few years, Yoga has found its way into the mainstream of American and Western society. Now, at the dawn of the twenty-first century, Yoga and its younger sibling, Power Yoga, are commonplace.

Yoga is now firmly embedded in Western culture. When you see a woman doing Yoga in a commercial, you know that Yoga has been mainstreamed. Everybody from athletes to health advocates, editors to celebrities (including Madonna and Sting — it's big with the one-name crowd) embrace Power Yoga.

Yoga is a five-thousand-year-old philosophy designed to promote a healthy physical, mental, and spiritual life. *Ashtanga Yoga* is the style of Yoga from which Power Yoga sprouted. Power Yoga takes the basics of Yoga and gives it a healthy dose of aerobics.

Imagine that — a system of Yoga that incorporates all the wonderful physical and mental benefits of Yoga and, in addition to toning all your muscles, gives you an aerobic workout and strengthens your heart — Powerful Yoga indeed!

Through the efforts of great American teachers like David Williams, Nancy Gilgoff, Norman Allen, David Swenson, Beryl Bender Birch, Brian Kest, and yours truly, Power Yoga has evolved into a popular Yoga alternative in the United States and other Western countries. I have tried my best to preserve their sincere integrity and compassion for Yoga in presenting you with this book, *Power Yoga For Dummies*.

You are not alone in your quest for Power Yoga. Many have discovered, as you will, that its benefits are endless.

Foolish Assumptions

For my part, I assume that you have heard of Yoga, know that it involves adopting certain poses, and are interested in finding out what Power Yoga can offer you. I don't assume much more.

For your part, please don't assume that Power Yoga is any less spiritual or relaxing than other forms of Yoga practiced today. Know that it involves adopting certain poses linked together with fluid, connecting links and that it can benefit you greatly.

How This Book Is Organized

Power Yoga For Dummies is divided into parts — seven of 'em. Each part addresses a different topic area and you can dip in and out of parts and chapters as the mood strikes you.

I organized the parts and chapters in a way that makes sense to me, but that doesn't mean that you have to read from cover to cover. In fact, I do my best to make it so that you don't have to. Of course, if you want to do one of the Power Yoga routines I offer, it helps to know the linking movements, or *vinyasas,* I set out in Chapter 10. But I provide lots of cross-references, so you can find out where I tell you how to do a pose or a *vinyasa.*

The information in this Introduction and the poses and other stuff on the Cheat Sheet give you all the tools you need to jump into a chapter, find a pose or routine you want to try, and just go for it.

I give you a rundown of what I put in each part to make it easier for you to find the information that interests you.

Part 1: Introducing Power Yoga Basics

These chapters concentrate on a general overview of Yoga and Power Yoga and how practicing Power Yoga engages your body and your mind.

Part 11: Preparing to Practice

In this part, I help you with the nuts and bolts of starting your Power Yoga practice. I give you pointers on how to incorporate Power Yoga into your daily routine. I tell you what you need in the way of special clothes and equipment (which isn't much) and where to find them. And I give you pointers on finding a Power Yoga teacher, from where to look to questions to ask a prospective instructor.

Part III: Mastering the Basics

The chapters in this part go through everything from basic poses to the linking movements unique to Power Yoga, as well as three complete Power Yoga routines — one each for beginning, intermediate, and advanced yogis and yoginis. Most of the illustrations in the book are in these chapters.

Part IV: Focusing on Specific Areas

If you want to target a specific fitness or body area, these chapters are for you. I offer exercises to improve your flexibility, strengthen your muscles, increase your endurance, and tone up your arms and abdominal muscles.

Part V: Enhancing Your Practice

The chapters in this part offer everything from advice on diet and nutrition (along with some yummy recipes) to practicing with a partner, as well as specific postures of benefit to women and seniors.

Part VI: The Part of Tens

In this traditional *For Dummies* part, I give you ten reasons to get into Power Yoga, ten tips for getting the most from your practice, and my ten favorite outdoor practice places.

Part VII: Appendixes

In Appendix A, you can find the Sanskrit terms for Yoga poses. And Appendix B lists Yoga and Power Yoga resources, including books, magazines, videotapes, and Web sites, as well as info on where to get your Yoga accessories.

Conventions Used in This Book

I try to keep the jargon to a minimum, so if you're brand-new to Power Yoga or Yoga in general, you can still understand what I'm talking about. However, I do use some Yoga and Power Yoga terms that you'll encounter if you expand your interest in Yoga or Power Yoga even a little beyond this book.

Eyeing those icons

All Dummies books use these handy icons to give you a heads-up about particular information. In *Power Yoga For Dummies,* I use these:

Power Yoga accommodates folks at various levels of ability and fitness. This icon points out alternative ways to do a pose — usually an easier way, or one that incorporates a prop.

Sanskrit is the original language of Yoga, and I provide the Sanskrit terms for most of, if not all, the poses and concepts I talk about. This icon lets you know when I do this.

Information next to this icon is good to keep in mind during a specific exercise or routine — sometimes throughout your Power Yoga practice.

When I share knowledge I've gained throughout my years of Yoga and Power Yoga practice or give you hints about how to achieve a specific pose or goal, I drop this icon next to it.

Vinny is a super Power Yogi who alerts you to information that puts the *power* in Power Yoga. His last name is the same as the linking movements that most obviously distinguish Power Yoga from traditional Yoga.

Anytime you do physical activity without taking the proper care you risk injuring yourself. I put this icon next to information that tells you how to avoid undue strain or injury, or that tells you should avoid a particular posture altogether if you meet certain conditions.

This lightening bolt lets you know that this movement requires some of the power that Power Yoga is famous for.

Remember: Always check with your medical practitioner before embarking on a fitness program, especially if you have existing health issues.

Checking out other conventions

In addition to the icons, I use a couple more tricks to keep the text moving and your posing flowing.

Figuring out figures

Parts III and IV are packed with photographs illustrating the postures and linking movements I give instructions for. Because I don't have enough space to include a picture of a posture every time I use it, I put some of the most often-used poses on the Cheat Sheet at the front of the book.

I also refer you to poses and linking movements I explain in depth in a previous chapter, so knowing that I number figures consecutively in each chapter helps you refer back to them. So, if I say, "refer to Figure 10-9," you can flip to Chapter 10 and look at the ninth illustration. The caption beside each figure starts with the figure number, which makes finding a specific figure fast and fun. (Okay, maybe it's not that much fun, but using all those *F*s made me feel fantastic!)

Recognizing certain words

I draw your attention to Sanskrit words and to defined terms by *italicizing* them. Some of the Sanskrit terms I use a lot are:

- **Asana:** This means pose, posture, or position. I use all four of these words interchangeably, though I remind you what *asana* means the first time I use it in a chapter.

- **Vinyasa:** One of the most obvious differences between Yoga and Power Yoga is that Power Yoga incorporates linking movements, or *vinyasas*, between poses for a fluid, flowing routine that keeps your body moving and your blood pumping. I add this definition at least once in the chapters I use it in, but I also use it frequently on its own.

- **Bandha:** This translates as "muscle lock," and I often tell you to engage different locks as part of a pose or linking movement. I talk more about the various *bandhas* in Chapter 7, and I show you where they're located both in that chapter and on the Cheat Sheet at the front of the book.

- **Prana:** Prana is the vital life force that everyone taps into. In Power Yoga, you focus on accepting and strengthening this energy.

You can also check the first appendix at the back of the book for definitions (and often the pronunciation) of Yoga and Sanskrit terms I use in this book.

Where To Go from Here

If you want to get the basics, start with the chapters in Part I. If you want to take care of the logistics before practicing, go to Part II. If you're anxious to get going and have some Yoga experience, head for the routines in Parts III and IV. If you need some motivation to get going, check out Chapter 23 in the Parts of Tens section.

In today's fast-paced society, the Earth often spins a bit too fast, making it difficult for your dreams and goals to keep pace. Power Yoga can help you find the middle way — the one that leads you to the best of all worlds.

Part I
Introducing Power Yoga Basics

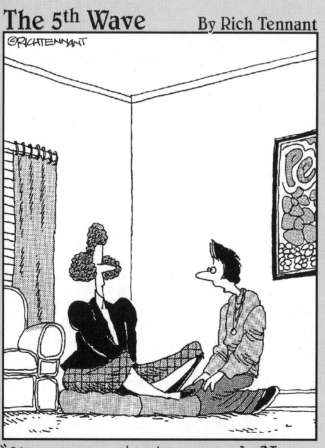

The 5th Wave   By Rich Tennant

©RICHTENNANT

"Okay, your posture's very good. Now relax, concentrate, and slowly let go of your cell phone."

In this part . . .

These chapters give you the basics. They tell you what Yoga is all about, and how Power Yoga developed from this centuries-old practice. I tell you what benefits you can expect not only physically, but mentally. So jump right in.

Chapter 1

Power Yoga in a Nutshell

For more than 5,000 years, people have been using the practice of Yoga to develop their mental, physical, and even spiritual well-being. But in the last decade or so, a revolution has taken place in this ancient practice, as Power Yoga has surged in the United States and around the world. Power Yoga combines traditional Yoga postures with fluid movements and key breathing techniques to deliver a powerful, nonstop aerobic workout. Power Yoga workouts are designed to maximize your power, energy, and vitality — and they deliver through a series of heart-thumping, sweat-pumping workouts that will leave you trim, energized, and heart healthy. Power Yoga gives your mind *and* body a powerful workout that you can customize to suit your athletic abilities and fitness goals. Whether you're a woman expecting a new Power-Yoga child, an on-the-go corporate executive trying to improve your physical and mental abilities, a senior citizen interested in maintaining — and even regaining — physical fitness, or a teenager interested in finding out more about Yoga practice, Power Yoga can be for you. This system is fully "customizable" to anyone's needs and is suitable for all ages, shapes, and sizes. You were especially smart to pick up this book, so you can start benefiting from Power Yoga in your life!

When I started practicing Yoga in 1968, I didn't have the opportunity to join a huge, thriving community of other yogis and yoginis. I had one or two good instructors of soft-form Yoga, but the practice of Power Yoga was yet undiscovered, and the road ahead for any practitioner was largely untraveled. You, on the other hand, are quite lucky to be starting your Power Yoga voyage today.

You have this book, so you have my 33 years of experience to help show you some ways to stay on a smooth path toward Power Yoga fitness. I can also help you avoid some of the potholes that I learned about through hard experience!

Whether you're 8, 18, or 80, Power Yoga can help you build a strong body, a clear mind, and a calm approach to life's daily dilemmas. In other words, Power Yoga is way cool, and so are those who practice it!

The best place to start your journey to Power Yoga nirvana is at the beginning. Find out what Power Yoga is all about, trace the path of Power Yoga from the ancient Indus Valley to your neighborhood fitness center, and see how Power Yoga can help you power up your life with style. Plug into the power!

Digging for the Roots of Power Yoga

The Sanskrit word *Yoga* can be translated to mean "union." *Yoga* is the union, integration, or balance of body, mind, and soul. Neither Richard Simmons nor Jane Fonda invented Power Yoga, and Madonna isn't the mother of the movement, either. Power Yoga is an offshoot of the practice of Yoga, which began thousands of years ago.

You can gain more benefits from the fruits of Power Yoga if you take a moment to study its roots, so help me start digging.

Finding the first Yogic sprouts

The first recorded evidence of Yoga dates to around 2500 B.C. and was discovered in an archaeological dig in India's Indus River Valley. Among the other remnants of an ancient, peaceful society, archaeologists uncovered a number of ancient stones engraved with drawings of people in Yoga poses. Like ancient trading cards, these Indus seals recorded the techniques and accomplishments of ancient *yogis* (practitioners of Yoga).

Building on the work of ancient masters

Very wise sages, who made the physical and mental well-being of mankind their ultimate goal, developed Yoga more than 5,000 years ago. The evolution of Yoga took the wisdom and thoughts of many generations. A pebble thrown in a pond makes ripples in the water, and that energy eventually touches every shore. In life, your existence creates ripples in time, like those in the pond. Because of the efforts of these sages many centuries ago, you and I feel the energy of Power Yoga expanding today.

It's all in the name

The language of Yoga — often taken from Sanskrit or Hindi — is beautiful and, in its own way, very precise. As in any discipline, the students and teachers of Yoga have specific names that indicate where they are in their ascent of the eight limbs of Yoga practice (see "Climbing the eight limbs of Ashtanga Yoga," later in this chapter):

A *yogi* is a male student of Yoga practice, though many people use the term to refer to any Yoga student, male or female. (Now that you've bought this book and are practicing Power Yoga, you can upgrade your status from dude to yogi.)

A *yogini* is a female student of Yoga practice. If you're a woman who's using this book to explore Yoga, why share a name with the guys? A beautiful flower deserves a beautiful name. You're a *yogini*.

A *Yoga master* is someone who has mastered the science, art, and practice of Yoga. We're all students and teachers, yet some practitioners reach incredible levels of achievement. These folks are the masters, and yogi and yogini pay respect to their awesome ability, achievement, and knowledge.

A *Brahmin* is a member of the elite, highest religious cast in Indian Hindu culture. Brahmins are usually well versed in sacred Yoga knowledge.

Ancient yogis lived and meditated in very close harmony with nature. The yogis carefully observed animals, birds, insects, and other forms of life, noting their postures, diets, and natural survival instincts. Using their observations, the early yogis developed a system of exercises, postures *(asanas)*, breathing practices, and philosophies that they hoped would benefit everyone. And what was the benefit? The achievement of *enlightenment*, a state of "oneness" with the universe, was the benefit. The yogis believed that enlightenment results in strength, inner peace, and understanding (both of yourself and the world around you).

While the Yoga masters were all working toward the same goal of achieving enlightenment, they actually developed different paths toward that goal; over time, these paths became specific types of Yoga. Jnana (pronounced *gyahnah*) Yoga, for example, has been called the Yoga of Wisdom, and it teaches that you gain enlightenment by gaining wisdom. Bhakti (pronounced *buhktee*) Yoga is called the Yoga of Devotion; practitioners believe that they achieve enlightenment by performing selfless acts of devotion.

Hatha (pronounced *huh-tuh*)Yoga is the Yoga of health and physical discipline. As such, it's sort of the grandmother of Power Yoga. Practitioners of Hatha Yoga believe that you must reach peak mental and spiritual condition in order to attain enlightenment. Practitioners of Hatha Yoga use postures and practices that are designed to get them into that peak physical *and* mental condition.

Hatha Yoga cleanses, strengthens, and purifies your body physically and mentally. This system uses a series of physical postures, breathing techniques, and cleansing exercises to teach practitioners discipline, confidence, willpower, and self-respect, and to build strength and flexibility while releasing stress and tension. Many of the postures and exercises you practice in this book sprang from Hatha Yoga.

Exploring the eight-limbed path

In 400 B.C., a wise sage and philosopher named Patanjali authored the oldest known Yoga text. Patanjali gathered the wisdom, experiences, and thoughts of many other Yoga teachers preceding him, along with teachings of his own, and created a book called *Yoga Sutras of Patanjali*.

Patanjali categorized the practice of Yoga into an eight-limbed path, designed to create balance and structure within the practice of Yoga. He divided the eight limbs into three categories of exercises and practice:

- ✔ **Ethical:** Practices that relate to abstinence, observance, and the study of moral and ethical codes to live by.

- ✔ **Physical:** Exercises that relate to postures, breath control, and the act of focusing the senses inward.

- ✔ **Mental:** Exercises that work to calm restless minds through techniques of concentration, meditation, and contemplation.

Patanjali's work is critical to the birth of the modern Power Yoga movement, because his teachings may have inspired its first form as a Yoga practice. To find out how Patanjali's work came to light, though, you have to fast-forward several hundred years, which I do in the "Exploring the eight-limbed path" section.

Climbing the eight limbs of Ashtanga Yoga

Ashtanga is a Sanskrit word that means "eight limbs." The eight limbs of Ashtanga Yoga are goals or aspects of yogic practice, through which you can reach the highest level of health and awareness.

- ✔ **Abstinence (Yama):** Moral guidelines to live by — being nonviolent, generous, trustworthy, truthful, and having integrity in your relationships.

- ✔ **Observances (Niyama):** Practices geared toward self-purification, including seeking purity of mind and body, seeking contentment or peace of mind, and practicing austerity, self-study, and attentiveness to God, or humble respect for the ultimate energy.

- **Posture *(Asana):*** Poses adopted during physical Yoga exercises that help to strengthen the body and increase willpower and self-confidence, resulting in a calm and relaxed mind.

- **Breath control (Pranayama):** The practice of using breath control to strengthen and direct the *prana* (life force) throughout your body. Practicing breath control improves your respiratory system, boosts concentration, helps to cleanse the body and mind, and revitalizes your immune system.

- **Sense withdrawal (Pratyahara):** The practice of withdrawing the mind from external concerns and stimuli and focusing it inward. Practicing sense withdrawal lets you ignore the noises around you, forget about the stresses of work and family, and take a break from worrying about bills and other energy-sappers. Sense withdrawal is essential for concentrating on the moment at hand.

- **Concentration (Dharana):** The practice of giving the full attention of your mind to a single idea or object. When you concentrate during Yoga practice, you give your full attention to the breathing, poses, and connecting *vinyasa* movements that make up your Yoga routine. Concentration is the bridge between the outside world and the world within your body.

- **Meditation (Dhyana):** A state achieved through the continuous flow of thought through concentration, awareness, and expansion of a thought or idea. When you meditate, you move one stage beyond concentration. In meditation, you don't have to work to keep your thoughts focused on a single idea; rather, you maintain a relaxed "gaze" upon some center focus. In this relaxed state of meditation, you really are observing your mind.

- **Contemplation (Samadhi):** A state of super-consciousness that you reach through continued meditation. Contemplation represents a state of peace and acceptance where you become one with all. It's the highest point you can reach in meditation and self-realization.

Tracking down the mother of Power Yoga

In the 1930s, a yoga master named Krishnamacharya and one of his most accomplished students, K. Pattabhi Jois, a Brahmin from Mysore, were doing some research in India at the Calcutta University library. During their research, they discovered an ancient document written in Sanskrit on palm leaves and bound like a manuscript. This document, written by Vamana Rishi, was about 1,500 years old and became known as the *Yoga Korunta* (ancient document or book, later known as Ashtanga Yoga, the mother of Power Yoga). Many scholars believe the Yoga Korunta is connected with the teachings of Patanjali.

Visiting the boys from India

Some of the world's most highly respected and influential Yoga masters lived in Mysore, India. If not for the efforts of this "Mysore Connection," the world would still be in Yoga's dark ages. Give your highest respect to the following Yoga masters:

✔ **Krishnamacharya** was born in 1890; he was a Sanskrit scholar and one of the most highly respected Yoga masters of modern times. Co-founder of the study of the legendary Yoga Korunta, (ancient documents discovered in 1930's, later known as Ashtanga Yoga) Krishnamacharya taught an individualized style of Yoga that catered to each student's particular needs. He died in 1989 at the age of 100.

✔ **K. Pattabhi Jois** was born in 1915. He is a Yoga master, Sanskrit scholar, and founder of Ashtanga Yoga. He studied with Krishnamacharya for many years. Jois is a very calm and passive man, who was still teaching Yoga at an advanced age.

✔ **B.K.S. Iyengar** was born in 1918 and is an accomplished Yoga Master and student of Krishnamacharya. Iyengar was greatly responsible for the popularity of Yoga in America. In 1966, he published a classic Yoga text, "*Light on Yoga*," and opened Yoga centers all over the United States. Iyengar originally practiced *vinyasa*-style Yoga (which has connecting links) but has adopted a style that incorporates the use of props and is very strict on *asana* (Yoga posture) alignment.

✔ **Desikachar** is the son of Krishnamacharya and studied with his father for about 30 years. His style, called *Viniyoga*, is much like his father's in that he takes an individual approach to teaching his students.

The Yoga Korunta described a system of Yoga that used fluid linking movements, called *vinyasa,* to connect Yoga postures into one seamless exercise. The Yoga Korunta included detailed instructions, written in rhyming phrases, on how to enter and exit each Yoga posture. This system was designed to promote physical and mental rejuvenation, peace of mind, and spiritual enlightenment. In later years, Jois became recognized as a master of this new system of Yoga and began teaching it in India. He named the system Ashtanga Yoga. Think of Ashtanga as the mother of Power Yoga.

Giving Birth to Power Yoga

By the 1960s, Yoga had become a small movement in the United States. In the decade that followed, Hollywood folks and East Coast intellectuals adopted it as an important technique to attaining physical and spiritual well-being. As Yoga gained popularity in the United States, the different types of Yoga began to separate into two major categories — soft and hard.

Up until the 1980s, most of the Yoga taught in America was of the soft form: Sivananda and Integral Yoga, for example. Soft-form Yoga practice emphasizes meditation, relaxation, and separate, distinct postures. Soft-form Yoga takes little energy and doesn't rely on high-energy physical workouts to achieve physical, mental, and spiritual health.

Ashtanga is a prime example of hard-form Yoga, in that it emphasizes attaining physical strength, improving muscle action, and building physical vitality and endurance. Unlike the slow, studied movements of most soft-form Yoga practices, Ashtanga relies on nonstop, high-energy routines that increase the circulation, raise body heat, and get your heart and lungs working.

Yoga is all about balance. You should consider incorporating both hard-form and soft-form Yoga practices into your life. In this book, I structure the routines to include both forms of Yoga so you can find the balance that's best for you and your lifestyle.

Powering up the United States

In the mid-1970s, Ashtanga Yoga was being taught in a few Yoga centers on the East and West Coasts, by early Ashtanga practitioners, such as Norman Allen, David Williams, and David's wife, Nancy Gilgoff. Over the next several years, Ashtanga Yoga gained popularity. Even so, by the late 1980s, Ashtanga Yoga was the practice of only a small percentage of the Yoga population.

In 1981, Beryl Bender Birch walked into Norman Allen's Ashtanga Yoga class in New York City and was absolutely convinced that she had found her true path in life. Beryl had studied numerous styles of Yoga in centers around the United States, but immediately knew she had found what she was looking for with Ashtanga. After many years of intensive study with Norman Allen and Pattabhi Jois himself, Beryl decided to begin teaching Ashtanga Yoga.

By the late 1990s, Beryl and her husband, Thom Birch, were among many teachers who were promoting the concept of Ashtanga Yoga.

In 1995, Beryl and Thom released a book called *Power Yoga* to convey the benefits of their increasingly distinct form of Ashtanga Yoga practice. The book was a smashing success and helped create a surge of interest in Power Yoga. People rushed to embrace the idea of losing weight, building strength, and enjoying an aerobic workout, all within the calming and spiritual framework of Yoga practice.

Taking a look inside the Power Yoga toolkit

Power Yoga makes use of a number of special tools — some are physical objects, some are mental states, some are specific types of movement, and others are a combination of the three. I give you the lowdown on all these tools in Chapter 7, but here's a sneak preview:

✔ **Asana:** One of the eight limbs of Ashtanga Yoga, these are the postures or poses you assume during Power Yoga practice.

✔ **Bandha:** These are muscular contractions or "locks" used to direct vital life-force energy *(prana)* throughout your body and to give your Power Yoga postures stability.

✔ **Body heat:** This is the term I use to describe the high-energy output state you reach in your Power Yoga workout; when you've attained high body heat, your breathing is fast, your heart and lungs are pumping, and you're probably sweating!

✔ **Drishti:** These are gazing points that you focus on as you assume various postures and movements during your routine; drishti help you draw your senses inward so you can concentrate on the effects of the *asana* you are performing.

✔ **Pranayama:** Also one of the eight limbs of Ashtanga Yoga, this carefully studied practice of controlled breathing helps you increase vital life-force energy throughout your body as you work out. Controlled breathing helps boost the flow of oxygenated blood throughout your body and leads to a more effective workout.

✔ **Props:** Pillows, blocks, straps, supports, and mats can help you comfortably assume some poses.

✔ **Vinyasa:** These connecting movements keep your body moving, your heart and lungs working, and your body heat high as you switch from one *asana* to the next.

Breaking away: Power Yoga finds its own identity

Over the last few years, the practices of Power Yoga and traditional Ashtanga Yoga have become clearly distinct, and today the two typically are taught as separate practices. I endorse both Power Yoga and Ashtanga Yoga and think they're both excellent practices.

The differences between the two Yoga practices are subtle and can depend (to a certain degree) on each teacher's intentions and individual training. Generally, the types differ in these ways:

Ashtanga Yoga (also known as Astanga), as taught in the traditional form of K. Pattabhi Jois, involves rules that are less flexible than those of Power Yoga. Ashtanga Yoga requires a specific (and unchanging) order of posture sequence. This order is maintained to help preserve the integrity of the ancient system, which may or may not seem worthwhile to you, depending on your level of practice. Traditional Ashtanga caters to young, more-athletic types, and it can be really difficult for people who don't have any previous experience in Yoga. On the upside, practicing Ashtanga immerses you in a very pure strain of Yoga practice, and it can get you in shape quickly.

Power Yoga isn't quite as regimented as the Ashtanga Yoga, so it caters to a wider group of students. The order of postures in Power Yoga can change, allowing the teacher and student room for creativity. As a result, Power Yoga lets you choose from an assortment of alternative routines, depending upon your mood and your level of fitness. The concept is based on the teachings of K. Pattabhi Jois, flavored with a strong influence from the teachings of the ancient master Patanjali's Yoga Sutras. In many ways, Power Yoga represents an American version of Ashtanga Yoga.

Power Yoga helped take Yoga instruction into the mainstream of modern life. Today, you can find Power Yoga teachers in health clubs, dance studios, college classes, and Yoga centers. Power Yoga has become one of the most popular Yoga practices, as people of all ages and interests have discovered its many benefits.

So what are you waiting for?

Realizing the Benefits of Power Yoga

Many people approach Power Yoga at its most basic level, as a physical fitness training program. Power Yoga delivers a powerhouse workout through its combination of breathing, stretching, muscle toning, aerobics, and deep relaxation techniques. In Power Yoga routines, you don't stop the action between postures, rest a moment, and then assume a new pose. The *vinyasas* (linking poses) that connect Power Yoga postures keep you active and moving. And the breathing techniques and mental focus you use throughout the routine keep your energy level high, so you get the most from every Power Yoga posture.

So Power Yoga, with its full aerobic workout, *is* a great fitness program — but it's also much more. Practicing Power Yoga is also a great way to achieve self-awareness; it can enhance your physical, mental, and spiritual health. In other words, it's a total approach to fitness.

In addition to its hard-body, high-energy workouts and exercise routines, this book delivers lots of helpful information on incorporating meditation, diet, and Yoga-friendly lifestyle patterns into your regular Power Yoga practice. In other words, *Power Yoga For Dummies* dishes up a large helping of power, with a tasty side of freedom and creativity.

Take a closer look at some of the ways that Power Yoga can work to get your entire self into great shape.

Pumping up your body with Power Yoga

Everybody gets something unique from Power Yoga practice, but most people are drawn to Power Yoga for the big gains in physical fitness that it offers. You can use Power Yoga to help you accomplish the following:

✔ **Strengthen your muscles:** The Power Yoga postures strengthen and stretch your muscles, and the aerobic workout builds your heart. (Don't forget *that* important muscle!)

✔ **Increase your flexibility:** Your muscles, joints, and tendons gain both strength *and* flexibility through the combined impact of Yoga postures, the *vinyasa* connecting movements, and Power Yoga's aerobic boost to your heart rate and metabolism.

✔ **Improve your endurance:** The nonstop Power Yoga workout, including postures, *vinyasas,* and controlled breathing techniques, delivers a high-energy routine that boosts physical endurance.

✔ **Lose weight (the big kahuna):** Power Yoga has become so popular because people discovered how successfully it melts off excess weight. Practitioners lose both pounds and inches as they burn calories and fat while firming muscles.

Sharpening your mind with Power Yoga

Losing weight, boosting your metabolism, and becoming stronger and more flexible — these are some very attractive reasons for practicing Power Yoga. But don't forget that 5,000-year-old central goal of all Yoga practice: the achievement of enlightenment. Power Yoga works toward that goal, too, by helping you achieve greater physical *and* mental power.

Remember that *enlightenment* refers to the act of becoming one with the universe — and with your own spiritual nature. Suppose that you reach enlightenment through this book. You'll rise above ego and be able to view life as a whole, unlimited by the confining perspective of the human body. In the Indian culture, the word for this state of mind is *atman* (pure consciousness), which is the threshold to *samadhi* (self-realization), the highest stage of Yoga meditation.

Through regular practice of Power Yoga, you can climb all eight limbs of Ashtanga Yoga (see "Climbing the eight limbs of Ashtanga Yoga" earlier in this chapter) and achieve a number of physical *and* mental benefits. I list just some of the good things that Power Yoga does for your head here:

- ✔ **Releases stress and tension:** Practicing Yoga postures, combined with deep breathing, helps relieve stress.

- ✔ **Calms and relaxes your mind:** You'll find relaxation through inverted Yoga poses, breathing techniques, concentration, and meditation.

- ✔ **Improves your concentration:** As stress and tension melt away and you practice the postures and breathing techniques, you can achieve deep relaxation. These benefits combine to increase your powers of concentration.

- ✔ **Helps you think outside the box:** Power Yoga teaches you to expand your thoughts and your mind; to see things, people, and their actions in context; and to draw upon all your mental resources in evaluating issues and finding solutions.

Feeding your soul with Power Yoga

Power Yoga is a tool that you can use to improve every aspect of your daily life, whether you're a scientist, fast-food employee, student, or whatever. This system gives you self-confidence and strength as it relieves stress and tension. Power Yoga can help you find peace and contentment. You may even find that it gives you a whole new appreciation for life — and that can be a benefit for you and everyone who knows you.

Power Yoga has become a popular practice because of the internal benefits. People want to be more in touch with themselves and with the world around them. In today's society, you get up and follow your fellow humans to work and rush through your daily activities. You spend most of the day around people and *doing* something, but most of the time you aren't really connected to the people or activities that make up your life. Power Yoga puts you in touch with your world and helps you be *of* it, not just *in* it. Power Yoga can improve how you interact with your world in these ways:

- ✔ **Hear as well as listen.** Through Power Yoga, you discover how to listen to other people and actually *hear* what they really say to you. As a bonus, you retain more of the true meaning of their words.

- ✔ **See with insight and clarity.** Power Yoga helps you to register the things that are before your eyes and to recognize what you're seeing. You see clearly, with your heart as well as your eyes, using insight and compassion.

- ✔ **Find peace of mind.** By lowering your heart rate, smoothing your respiratory process, and calming your mind, Power Yoga helps you be calm and at peace with the world.

These benefits are something that everyone, not just a few Yoga masters, can achieve. You can enjoy these three important benefits through regular Power Yoga practice, body cleansing, meditation, and deep relaxation techniques.

Putting the Power to Your Yoga

The previous sections tell you how Power Yoga can serve to greatly enhance your self-awareness and daily existence by creating a union of body and mind, and how you can use Power Yoga to build strength, gain self-confidence and awareness, and even improve your ability to communicate with others in your life. So how do you incorporate Power Yoga into your daily routines? I tell you how in the following sections.

The busier your life is, the more you can benefit from adding a soothing touch of Power Yoga to your routine. Luckily, getting started in Power Yoga is easy. You can start off with a practice of 20 to 30 minutes, two or three times a week. Morning and evening are the most tranquil times for practice; however, any time will do. Pick a routine from this book (see Part III) that seems most appropriate for your present level of fitness. Find a quiet, clean, warm space, and give it a try. Always allow a few minutes after practice to lie down and relax. In a week or so, you'll start feeling all the wonderful benefits of Power Yoga. As your body gets in better shape, you can sample the more challenging workouts I provide, and you may even want to start creating your own Power Yoga routines. You may even want to add more days to your practice schedule, too. It's your gig, so make it work for you.

Power Yoga can bring you some benefits, whether you choose to practice it as a daily, every-other-day, or semi-weekly exercise routine, or adopt it as a way of life. Living a Power Yoga lifestyle involves more than sweating it out through an exercise program; true Power Yoga practitioners know that its benefits are connected like links in a chain. As you become stronger and more flexible, you become more relaxed and calm. You begin to care more about yourself and the world around you. As a result, you take better care of your body *and* your world — and both your body and your world benefit.

You can choose to *do* Power Yoga and gain some benefits from it, or you can choose to *live* Power Yoga and achieve even more.

No one area of mastery can help you gain the maximum benefit from Power Yoga. You really have to work on the entire package. As a student of Power Yoga, for example, you should strive to preserve the great lessons of the past and, at the same time, incorporate your own creative knowledge of physical and mental stamina and fitness techniques. And don't forget to embrace the power, beauty, and knowledge of nature within your body and mind.

Throughout this book, I show you many Power Yoga postures and routines that you can use to build your mastery of Power Yoga as you work toward your fitness goals. After you become familiar with your Power Yoga practice, I bet you'll want to create your own routines so you can put together a program that best fits your lifestyle. Feel free to create! That's what Power Yoga is all about.

Working the Power Yoga system for all it's worth

Power Yoga has all the benefits of traditional soft-form Yoga, yet you also receive an aerobic and anaerobic workout. This enables you to get in great shape, and to gain flexibility and find total deep relaxation.

The whole system of Power Yoga is based on becoming more aware of the connection among your body, mind, and soul. After you find your balance between *yin and yang* (the opposing life forces), you can surf your *prana* energy and glide through life like a surfer riding a wave in the ocean.

Fueling your body with energy to burn

You become more aware of your body through regular Power Yoga practice. That increased awareness is likely to make you more concerned about the fuel that you use to keep your body going. The more demands you make on your body, the more important your diet becomes. Turn to Chapter 22 for some easy-to-follow guidelines for a healthy, natural diet that can help you get the most from your Power Yoga practice. In the beginning, I encourage you to strive for simple changes in your diet. Maybe you can begin by staying away from sugar for a few meals, and then you can slowly add more fresh foods and fiber to your diet.

Reading about diet and nutrition isn't much fun, though, if you don't have some good recipes to back up the advice. Don't worry! You can go crazy with the recipes for Power smoothies and monkey shakes that I provide in Chapter 22. These high-energy, great-tasting drinks give you energy and nutrition to burn — without demanding that you also burn off lots of empty calories!

Powering up with a friend

Although Power Yoga can be highly individualized, it's not something you have to do alone. Through Power Yoga practice, you'll probably meet lots of new friends. And you may decide to share your Power Yoga practice with family or co-workers. Partner work is an extremely helpful and fun way to practice Power Yoga.

In Part VI, I list a few of my favorite Yoga adjustments along with some creative partner poses. Partnered Power Yoga is definitely one of the most fun ways to practice, and it can bring an excellent boost to your skill in attaining the Yoga postures. In the Power Yoga world, if you make a hands-on correction for another Yoga student, you're doing what's called an *adjustment,* an act that can greatly assist anyone in finding the right posture alignment. Your partner can make adjustments for you, too, which will help move you toward the goal of mastering the postures and connecting moves.

Adding all the right moves to other Yoga practices

If you are presently practicing a "softer" style of Yoga, you're in a great position to move on up to Power Yoga. You can try stepping up the power a bit by introducing *vinyasas* (those all-important connecting links) between the Yoga postures that you currently practice. When you tie poses together with connecting movements, you're essentially creating power lines that keep the energy moving between Yoga postures — just like electrical power lines keep energy flowing between cities. I show you how to do this in later chapters, as well.

Power Yoga doesn't require that you move really fast, like you do in aerobics or dance classes. Just hold a steady pace with powerful breathing attached to your movements. I know you will be delighted with the result and find power surging throughout your body and mind.

Personalizing your Power Yoga practice

Power Yoga encourages practitioners to be really creative in finding new and creative ways to practice. In the following list, I suggest ways to personalize your Power Yoga practice:

- ✔ **Enjoy Yoga with the soothing touch of nature.** If you've never practiced Yoga outdoors, you are in for a real treat. Your Power Yoga practice is given a huge boost by the magic of nature — it can be the ultimate natural high! When you sit on the ground, watch the gentle rhythm of the flowers dancing in the wind, and feel the energy from a mighty oak, you can truly say, "This is living!"

- ✔ **Practice power routines to enhance athletics.** I've been a major sports and recreation buff for years, and I know that Power Yoga has helped me greatly improve my balance, strength, and speed.

- ✔ **Create your own personal yoga routine.** You're a creative person (or you soon will be!). So don't be afraid to use your natural creative drive to craft your own fun Power Yoga routines.

You can adapt Power Yoga any number of ways — it's a very flexible discipline.

Chapter 2

Powering Up Your Body

. . . .

In This Chapter

▶ Making it *all* good with Power Yoga

▶ Strengthening your machine

▶ Detoxifying your lungs

▶ Getting your blood flowing

. . . .

Power Yoga practice has a dramatic effect on your whole body — inside and out, from your head to your toes. In fact, the dramatic fitness benefits of Power Yoga attract many practitioners in the first place; discovering the many other benefits of a Power Yoga lifestyle can be an added bonus!

This chapter focuses on fitness. I clue you in on how to make the most of your Power Yoga practice, which can enhance everything from your skin tone to your respiratory health. And I show you how to use Power Yoga to get even better at the sports and recreational activities you know and love. So get ready to take a quick peek inside your anatomy and find out all the ways that Power Yoga can boost your body — on both sides of its skin!

Upgrading Your Anatomy

Power Yoga affects literally every aspect of your anatomy — your muscles, bones, and respiratory and circulatory systems — and the way those elements work together. Practicing Power Yoga postures *(asanas)* stretches your muscles and aligns your skeletal framework with its tendons and ligaments. The breathing techniques of Power Yoga help keep your respiratory system working efficiently, which dramatically aids your circulation. When you breathe more effectively, your heart has to do less work. And the linking movements that you do to connect each posture help you maintain a powerful, aerobic pace that gives your whole body a full-fledged power workout.

Teachers and experienced practitioners of Power Yoga believe that each Power Yoga routine benefits your body in different ways. They call the postures designed to aid specific parts of your body *curative asanas* because they have experienced or seen these postures make real and lasting changes, either in themselves or in their students. For example, some Power Yoga postures help align your spinal column, while others improve the functions of your heart, liver, or thyroid gland (which all affect your energy levels). As you become more familiar with Power Yoga postures and their benefits, you can design personalized routines to include curative *asanas* to work on the aspects that you want to improve.

And finally, Power Yoga works to benefit your anatomy through its boost to your circulatory system. Throughout this book, I make frequent references to "internal heat" and "body heat." Don't worry — I've never known anyone to burst into flames from a Power Yoga workout! These terms simply refer to the increased heart rate and circulation that you achieve when you move through a Power Yoga routine. When you sweat during a routine, your body is getting the incredible benefit of Power Yoga delivered directly to and through your circulatory system. It's a great way to get an aerobic workout, and you know how important this is to your cardiovascular health. The more pumped up you get, the more body heat you generate. As you discover later in this chapter, body heat is a good thing in Power Yoga.

Your body benefits from your practice of Power Yoga in three primary ways:

- From practicing curative poses
- From practicing *pranayamas*, or proper breathing techniques
- By improving your circulatory system through *asanas* and connecting movements, or *vinyasas*

Take a closer look at each of these benefits and how you can achieve them.

Getting in Line with Curative Asanas

The Sanskrit word *asana* means "seat," "posture," or "position." *Asanas* are the core of nearly every form of Hatha Yoga practice, including Power Yoga. Curative Yoga *asanas* are designed to restore and rejuvenate your total physical and mental health. These postures keep the body strong and in tune with nature.

The system of Yoga *asanas,* developed over thousands of years, systematically stretches, tones, strengthens, and relaxes every aspect of your body. Power Yoga routines include numerous *asanas* that involve forward bending, backward bending, and twisting movements. Some Yoga postures require that you stand upright, while others may have you hanging upside down! The ordering of the *asanas* is specifically designed to deliver the maximum rejuvenating effect. You can use curative *asanas* (Yoga postures designed to help relieve physical and mental problems throughout your body) to help your body in these ways:

Looking into the benefits of gazing

To get the most from your Yoga *asanas,* use a technique called the drishti. The *drishti* is a gazing point — some object or point in space on which you focus your gaze as you assume and hold each pose. Focusing on a specific point helps you draw your senses inward to concentrate on the posture you've assumed and the way your body feels in that posture.

Power Yoga uses gazing to help you, in effect, keep an eye on your anatomy during practice — to help you maintain your body's alignment, hold a muscle lock, or continue a breathing technique. Maintaining proper breathing techniques is another way to benefit your body during Power Yoga. Easy breathing links the physical movements and mental concentration that are essential to a good Power Yoga practice. Breathing is easy, but *easy* breathing, or *ujjayi* breathing, takes a bit of practice. I talk more about that in the section "Breathing Easy with Pranayamas " in this chapter.

✔ **Correct skeletal alignment:** Your skeletal alignment affects the way you walk, your posture, how you perform at work or at play, and even how you relax. Whether you spend your days at work, in school, or simply enjoying normal recreation and leisure activities, many common daily activities can subtly shift your skeletal framework out of alignment. For example, if you lift something too quickly or from the wrong position, one of your spinal vertebrae may shift out of proper alignment.

Everybody has a posture no-no — I round my shoulders, and you may lift with your back instead of your legs. The good news is that you can correct these misalignments by practicing curative Yoga *asanas.* And by merely doing the poses, you help restore balance to your muscles. The side benefit is that, as you become more aware of your everyday posture, you can tap into the feel of a curative *asana* to help correct it.

✔ **Limber up joints, tendons, and ligaments:** A very healthy man named Paul Bragg, who died at age 99 while body surfing in Hawaii, once said, "To rest is to rust." You have to use your joints to keep them in proper working order. Power Yoga is designed to strengthen your joints, helping to keep them lubricated, healthy, and functioning properly. Joints stiffen with age, and Power Yoga actually helps to reverse this part of the aging process by rejuvenating your joints. If you practice moderate Power Yoga on a regular basis, you can maintain your youthful flexibility of tendons, ligaments, and joints throughout your life.

✔ **Strengthen muscles:** Many other forms of physical fitness strengthen muscles, but they don't give proper attention to helping your body accommodate those stronger muscles. Your muscles tighten as you work them; over a period of weeks, this tightness can cause the muscles to shorten and become extremely tense. This tension can make you prone to injury, and it can also be very uncomfortable. In Power Yoga, you work your muscles to help them become firm, but you also stretch the muscles equally in all directions. This technique leaves your muscles strong, yet relaxed and free from tension.

✔ **Rejuvenate your endocrine system:** The endocrine system is a network of organs and tissues in the body that secrete hormones directly into the bloodstream. Anyone who remembers puberty and its associated hormonal "swings" can attest to the fact that hormones have a great effect on your emotions. The systematic practice of curative Yoga *asanas* gives your endocrine glands an internal massage that serves to keep these glands in proper working order. By helping to keep your endocrine system healthy, Power Yoga can work to help you avoid mood swings, depression, and anxiety.

Breathing Easy with Pranayamas

Okay, you already know how to breathe, right? But maintaining proper Yoga breathing is one of the most important aspects of your Power Yoga practice. When you're first born, you get slapped on the caboose to start your breathing, and when you die, that long exhale is the last thing you do. Because breathing is essential for life, mastering proper breathing techniques can have a huge impact on the quality of the life you live.

In Yoga, the vital life force is called *prana. Prana* is energy that emanates from all the elements of life — earth, air, fire, water, and ether. You can channel the life-giving properties of these elements through your body by controlled breathing — a practice known as *pranayama*. Think of pranayama as a way to extract concentrated life energies from the air around you, just as a juice extractor extracts concentrated vitamins and minerals from fruits and vegetables. In an analogous process, pranayama helps you get all the life-giving "juice" from oxygen and deliver it throughout your body, where it's transformed into power, strength, and relaxation.

Power Yoga's breathing techniques can help your whole respiratory system in these and other ways:

Breathing best

To get the most from your Power Yoga practice, make sure that you set the stage for following the proper breathing techniques. Practice in a clean environment with plenty of fresh air in the room. If the room's a bit stuffy, try filling it with plants — they release oxygen, filter the air, and help the place look better, too. Better yet, practice Power Yoga outdoors, where fresh air is freely available — unless you're next to the freeway, in which case, go back to your plant-filled room.

✔ **Increasing your lung capacity:** Power Yoga teaches you to inhale and exhale slowly and completely; after you've practiced this way of breathing over a period of months, you can actually expand the capacity of your lungs. In practicing traditional exercise methods, you may not breathe in enough oxygen to compensate for the energy you burn, which can leave you with sore muscles, tension, stress, and a lack of energy. In Power Yoga, your expanded lung power pulls in more oxygen with each breath, so you're feeding your brain, blood, and muscle tissue the oxygen they need to work hard. As a result, you have abundant energy coming from the oxygenated blood that pumps through your body.

✔ **Cleansing your respiratory system:** As you continue to do your slow, deep Power Yoga breathing, you'll cleanse smoke, pollution, and other toxins from your lungs. Short inhalations and exhalations can leave pollutants trapped in the lungs; the deep, complete breathing in Power Yoga can help saturate the lungs with fresh oxygen each time you breathe in, and then can flush toxins out of the lungs as you completely exhale.

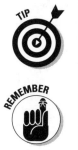

Power Yoga breathing techniques give you a tool for warding off colds and flu. Power Yoga can't cure the common cold, but it can aid your system in avoiding one. Some pranayama exercises, practiced at the beginning and end of your Power Yoga routines, can help you further target healthy respiratory function.

✔ **Increasing your vital life force:** Imagine a candle burning in a jar; if you put a top over the jar, the flame burns weaker and then dies as it consumes the oxygen in the jar. If you supply abundant of fresh oxygen to the flame, it burns strong and vibrant. Think of your own vital life force (or *prana*) as being much like that burning flame. If you do not take in abundant oxygen through regular active Yoga, your energy and vital life force are oxygen-starved and weakened. If you are very sick, your vital life force is weak. If you are strong and have robust energy, your vital life force burns strong. Through the practice of pranayama breathing techniques in Power Yoga, you stoke the furnace of your vital life force throughout your body.

✔ **Cultivating a tranquil mind:** When your emotions get a bit off-base and you feel upset or stressed out, your breathing is very short, choppy, and erratic. Slow, deep breathing techniques can actually calm your mind, relax you, and bring you greater peace. Power Yoga shows you how to use good breathing habits constantly — not just during your Power Yoga workouts — so you are constantly cultivating a calm and tranquil mind. These breathing techniques can be used in your daily life to help you stay centered while living in a stressful society.

Getting Your Blood Pumping

Your cardiovascular system keeps blood moving through your body in a process that seems to take no effort on your part, yet is essential to your life. The blood that circulates throughout your body helps to regulate your body temperature, and it carries oxygen to your brain, bone, muscle, and other tissue cells. Your circulatory system is also responsible for filtering and eliminating toxins from your body. If your circulatory system is strong and functioning properly, all is well, and your body's work gets done. If your circulatory system suffers, so do you.

Power Yoga's *vinyasa system* (a system linking Yoga postures together with a fluid movement) gives you a cardiovascular workout, speeds up your circulation, and strengthens your heart. You gain these benefits through light aerobic movements between the yoga poses *(vinyasas)*, combined with gentle stretching postures *(asanas)* and deep breathing techniques (pranayama). Power Yoga can work to improve the quality of your blood and circulatory system in these specific ways:

✔ **Avoiding and overcoming high cholesterol:** When cholesterol deposits clog your arteries, your heart has to pump harder to keep your blood flowing. Over time, fat deposits can completely block passages in your arteries, leading to strokes and heart attacks. By practicing Power Yoga regularly, you stretch, twist, massage, lengthen, and contract your veins and arteries, helping to prevent and break up cholesterol deposits. A strong, healthy flow of oxygenated blood helps to keep arterial walls clean; Power Yoga keeps blood pumping freely through your veins. Of course, stress, heredity, and diet are powerful factors in elevated cholesterol. Power Yoga is much more efficient at helping to keep your arteries clean and clear when you accompany the exercises with a healthy low-fat diet.

✔ **Strengthening your heart:** Your heart muscle circulates the blood throughout your body. If you don't get regular aerobic exercise, the heart muscle becomes weak and less efficient. (Did I mention that Power Yoga is a great aerobic workout?) Regular aerobic exercise helps to keep the heart healthy, strong, and functioning properly.

✔ **Creating easy blood flow:** With inverted Power Yoga postures, you help the heart distribute blood to the extremities of the body with less energy. Varicose veins are an adverse effect that you can experience if you spend long periods of time on your feet. By doing inverted Yoga postures, you put gravity to work for your heart, by helping it send blood to the extremities with less effort.

Okay, you believe that Power Yoga's poses, breathing techniques, and gazing can improve your flexibility, balance, energy levels, and concentration. But Power Yoga provides benefits in even subtler ways by boosting your confidence in your ability to manage new physical challenges. Just by sitting on your Yoga mat and trying new postures, you gain considerable confidence in your ability to master physical maneuvers. As the weeks roll by, Power Yoga teaches you to trust your body and know its limits. Your mind is clear and is working in strong connection with your body.

Chapter 3

Sharing Power with Your Mind

I'm sure that you know the saying, "A mind is a terrible thing to waste." Well, in Power Yoga, you don't waste a thing. Power Yoga helps you enhance your mind's many wonderful qualities and sharpen your mental clarity. Practicing Power Yoga also clues you in on ways to control your emotions, let go of stress, and get more in touch with the important relationships in your life. In this chapter, I show you how to use Power Yoga to tune up your mind at work, school, and play. You may be surprised at how Power Yoga helps you to improve your organizational skills, self-confidence, and the general efficiency of anything you do.

We all lose our cool now and then; that's just part of being human. In this chapter, you discover how the practice of Power Yoga helps you to keep these negative emotions under control, to find a balance between mind and body, and to spot "energy blocks" that prevent you from releasing stress. Finally, I show you how your Power Yoga practice can eliminate the problem in relationships that was summed up so well by the prison captain in *Cool Hand Luke* — "What we've got here is a failure to communicate." After you become more in touch with yourself through Power Yoga practice, you find that relating to friends, family, and lovers is much easier.

If you're just practicing Yoga on your exercise mat and not in your head, you aren't tapping into your full Power Yoga potential! So get ready for a mind-ful of Power Yoga.

Enhancing Your Mental Performance with "the Practice"

Power Yoga can seem like a magical gift for your mind. The rewards of Power Yoga practice are almost immediate, as you notice increased mental clarity, efficiency, and self-confidence. Even as it makes you more powerful, though, Power Yoga also cultivates the easy-going child within you. Your practice shows you what peace of mind really feels like and encourages you to kiss stress goodbye. The following sections take a closer look at some of the mental wonders that Power Yoga can work for you.

Meeting Mr. Clarity

Have you ever been in the mountains or along the coast on a very foggy summer morning? The fog can be so thick that the world seems to stop a few feet in front of you; you aren't sure where you are, and you can't see where you're going or where you've been. Then, in the afternoon, the fog lifts, and you see the wonderful colors of the trees, grass, wild flowers, and sky, and suddenly, you know exactly where you are in the landscape.

That same feeling of clarity and understanding can surround you after practicing Power Yoga. The fog lifts, and you see life much more clearly. Everything in your world seems greatly enhanced after a good Power Yoga session. The colors of flowers against the deep blue sky are more beautiful than usual; your work is more manageable, and you roll through your daily tasks more easily. And, you're better able to see things from all sides, not just from your own perspective.

The pause that powers

No matter how busy your day gets, try to make your Yoga practice the number one priority. It is hard to describe the feeling in your mind after Power Yoga practice: You're energized, yet relaxed; calm, yet very focused. If you start your day with a practice session, you can then shower, get dressed, and head out the door to tackle your list of daily chores with a light heart and a confident stride. You scratch off the last chore of the day in half the time that it usually takes to finish things, and you have energy left to take on more. Power Yoga isn't another daily grind; it's a way to take the grind out of your daily life.

Loving the fun in you

Hey, act your age! And whatever age you may be, you should feel free every now and then to let loose the playful child that lives within you. If you're totally serious all the time, you build up lots of tension. Being child-like is a healthy way to let go of that tension. I'm a great believer in the old notion that laughter is the best medicine, and it's especially good at relieving stress. So laugh and let your playful child appear now and then; you'll be happier, have more friends, live longer, and enjoy your own company.

 It's hard to deal with all the problems in life, but one good solution is to bend with the wind. Through practicing Power Yoga, you create a fluid, supple body, and in turn, you achieve a supple, calm, tranquil mind. But don't think that you have to sacrifice clarity to find tranquility! As a matter of fact, you'll find that your relaxed mind is quite clear and quick-on-the-draw.

Knowing that you can

 "Well, I'm just not sure; maybe I can, if things work out. Perhaps if you call me later, I may think about trying, but I don't think that I want to commit to anything right now." Sound familiar? Something as simple as self-confidence can make or break you in all areas of life, whether you're trying to get a job, ask someone out on a date, or survive a long walk across a desert. Power Yoga gives you the confidence you need to show a little backbone, stand up proud, and say, "Yes, I can!"

Your practice makes you stronger — physically and mentally. You gain the confidence you need to give life your best shot. With the support of a powerful system of Yoga backing you, you can use full power in all aspects of your life and ground yourself in nature for the firmest footing. Through your daily Yoga practice, you gain self-confidence as you discover new postures, focus your mind and energy, and feel the power of your control. This self-confidence has always been in you; Power Yoga just pulls it out of the storage bin for you to use.

Kissing stress goodbye, and finding peace of mind

 Think of stress as steam in a pressure cooker. As the stove's burner gets hotter, steam builds up in the pot and the pressure increases. If the cooker had no release valve to relieve the building pressure, the cooker would explode. The same is true with what happens to you in your daily life. As stress heats up your day, your tension grows and pressure builds; if you can't release some of the tension, you're liable to explode!

No matter how you sugarcoat it, you live in a stressful society, and getting caught up in the fast-paced confusion of today's world is easy. You can't avoid stress, but you can deal with it. Rather than exploding, you can use Power Yoga as your stress "release valve." Power Yoga is widely known as one of the best tools for releasing tension; a Power Yoga routine, followed by deep relaxation, brings a wonderful gift of peace of mind to your body and spirit.

Touching Your Emotions, and Feeling Your Creativity

Practicing Power Yoga generates enormous amounts of positive energy; this energy is stored as *prana* in your body and mind. *Prana* energy is the vital life-force energy taken into the body through the air that you breathe. This energy is contained within all the elements of life. As you practice Power Yoga, its *pranayama* (breathing techniques), *bandhas* (muscle locks), and *asanas* (postures) help you channel *prana* energy throughout your mind and body. Tapping into *prana* energy can make an amazing difference in your emotional state of being.

Through a regular Power Yoga practice, you can achieve the following:

- **Compassion for your fellow humans and all life:** When you practice Power Yoga, the fog that masks your true inner nature is lifted, and you can see and become more in tune with yourself. This self-knowledge also helps you view the world around you through the eyes of compassion; you gain respect and admiration for your fellow man and for Mother Nature.

- **A nonjudgmental attitude:** You know the saying, "Live and let live." Within the codes of ethics that a true yogi follows is the commitment to be non-judgmental in thought and action. You and I are neighbors on this planet with all kinds of folks from many cultures. The regular practice of Power Yoga helps you remember that a person's value in this world isn't determined by the car one drives, the food one eats, the lifestyle one lives, or the religion one follows — we're all equal under the sun. Yogis and yoginis extend the same respect to others that they expect to receive.

- **An open mind and creative perspective:** Yoga is about expanding your mind and cultivating your own creativity. Your Power Yoga practice helps you "think outside the box" and gives your own creativity a chance to grow and expand. Power Yoga can help you switch from tunnel vision to a panoramic view of the world around you, letting the sun shine in and illuminating the corners of your rich, creative mind. After you expand your own consciousness through Power Yoga practice, your creativity will soar.

The not-so-sweet nature of sugar

Along with your Power Yoga practice, you can greatly enhance your ability to control unstable emotions by limiting your intake of refined sugar and its byproducts. Refined sugars move quickly into your blood stream and release chemicals that can cause dramatic mood swings. And your body can become so fond of sugar that you crave it like an addict craves a drug. "Just saying no" to sugar can help you boost the mind- and body-building power of your Power Yoga practice.

Action without attachment is an important concept in Power Yoga. This concept demonstrates that you can get a job done efficiently and do what you have to do without letting your emotions get out of control. Panic, anger, disappointment, and sorrow are natural emotions; but when the time comes to act, you can achieve more by setting these emotions aside and moving forward with calm purpose through the task at hand. This kind of mental and emotional discipline is a natural side effect of Power Yoga practice.

Playing on the mood swing

Your emotions are your natural response to the people and situations that you encounter every day. How well you handle your emotions can determine how you get through your day and how you interact with those around you. Power Yoga practice is a key component for figuring out how to level off the ups and downs of mood swings.

Emotions are greatly affected by hormones, which your body can release quickly into your bloodstream in response to things happening around you. This surge of hormones can be a good thing if, for example, a lion is chasing you, and you need a quick burst of adrenaline to run to safety. It's bad, though, if a quick release of hormones causes you to fly off the handle at someone just because you had a bad day, and your nerves are on edge.

Power Yoga helps you build both mental and physical means for controlling the release of hormones throughout your body. If you view the people and things you encounter every day from a calm perspective, you limit that "knee-jerk" response that can make you and everyone around you nuts. Power Yoga's exercises can actually help you control the release of hormones into your blood stream. That ability combined with a calm, controlled mind are your best tools for taking the "swing" out of your emotional responses.

Watering your spiritual garden with Power Yoga

Often, I have been asked the question, "Is Yoga a religion or just a form of exercise?" This is a good question, and the answer is deceptively simple: Yoga can be both, or it can be neither. You decide what Yoga is for you — there are no ground rules in this area, and you have all the options in the universe. If you want to use Power Yoga for exercise, so be it. If you want to pursue an Eastern religion and practice Yoga as well, go for it. Though you don't have to follow any specific religion to practice Power Yoga, it's a fine way to water your spiritual garden.

Spirituality can mean different things to different people. For you, spirituality may mean being close to nature; to me, it's having a kind and generous heart; to another, it's showing compassion toward all creatures. In the same context, Power Yoga can bring you to whatever spiritual state you set out to achieve. If you practice Yoga in a peaceful atmosphere, are attentive to yourself, cultivate your mind-body connection, and feel the heartbeat of Mother Nature in your practice, Power Yoga can introduce you to the true spirituality within you. Whether you are religious or nonreligious, spiritual or not, Power Yoga can serve to increase your present beliefs, whatever those beliefs may be.

Warming up those cold thoughts

People have basically two categories of emotions: cold and negative or warm and positive. Examples of cold, negative emotions are hate, jealousy, anger, and deception. Examples of warm, positive emotions are joy, compassion, and love.

When you don't take care of your body properly, you damage your mental and emotional health, as well as your mental state. You probably have already discovered that when you don't exercise regularly, don't eat right, and don't get enough sleep, your body feels sluggish and run down.

But you may not have made the connection between how you function emotionally and your physical health. A poor physical condition makes you more likely to dwell on problems and obstacles, promoting negative emotional energy. This energy state promotes negative, defeatist attitudes and behavior. Thoughts are seeds: What you plant is what you grow. Negative thoughts grow into negative actions.

Enjoying Relationships with Power Yoga

One of the hardest things in life is communication; failures in this area can lead to friction between family members, separation between friends, and the death of loving relationships. And that's not even taking into account how many wars could have been avoided if communication between cultures had been healthy and alive.

Communication isn't the only key to strong relationships, of course. Healthy relationships are also made up of honesty, compassion, and loyalty — all held together by the glue of self-confidence that strengthens people and their relationships. Power Yoga can help you build these qualities in yourself and can assist you in forging stronger relationships with your family members, friends, and lovers.

Yoga can help you be better prepared, both mentally and physically, to deal with the ups and downs of any relationship. Working from a base of positive emotions, you develop a relaxed, rational state of mental clarity. Through practicing regular Yoga postures, breathing techniques, and deep relaxation methods, you can build a disciplined yet relaxed mind-body consciousness, which helps you communicate better and respond more compassionately to those around you.

Strengthening family ties

"Mammas, don't let your babies grow up to be Yogis! They're never at home, and they're always alone... "

Just kidding, mom! But the truth is, I'm on the road a lot, giving Power Yoga seminars and workshops around the country. I've seen up close and personal how Power Yoga can help maintain strong family relationships, even when circumstances don't seem to be favorable for a tight family bond.

Whether you are dealing with a life partner, brothers and sisters, parents and grandparents, or children and grandchildren, you must be able to talk to each other in a common vocabulary. That doesn't mean you have to say to your kids, "Like, I'm all, wow, totally cool, dude." I mean that you have to understand how each person in your family feels, see the world from his or her perspective, and deal with each person using the same kind of understanding and compassion that you want to receive from him. Power Yoga gives you the strength to do that.

Power Yoga can also boost your family ties in other ways: It can help you deal with the passing of a loved one, defuse conflicts among family members, and relax enough to enjoy your family life. Again, your emotional state greatly affects your relationships; Power Yoga helps to stabilize your emotional state so you can develop better bonds with the whole family.

Forming true friends

I'm sure that you've heard it said often, but let me repeat it: Friends are truly a priceless gift and not something to be taken for granted. Power Yoga gives you a big boost in body and spirit that helps you enjoy the time you spend with your friends and helps others enjoy *you* more, too. People love to be around yogis and yoginis because they exude wonderful, positive, up-beat energy. You're more fun to be around, and you have extra energy throughout the day when you're practicing Power Yoga. You develop a more relaxed state of mind, a self-confident attitude, and a well-grounded approach to life. These qualities are helpful when you're interacting with friends.

Making the most of your love relationships

Powering Up Your Love Machine

Dreams often lend themselves to paradise

As the days play out the past;

Yet, of all the pleasures in life,

Memories of your smile will always last.

Love is what life's all about, and as my poem indicates, I think that true love benefits you forever — maybe even after the love affair has ended. Power Yoga, with all its physical, mental, and spiritual benefits, is a powerful force in every aspect of your "good loving" approach to life.

Power Yoga tones up your entire body. With regular Power Yoga practice, you begin to notice higher sensual vibrations and better communication with your partner, which both lead to more powerful lovemaking. Power Yoga practice shows you compassion, focus, and clarity, and it can serve to heighten your senses. You see more clearly and touch with every fiber of your body; you are in complete contact with your emotions. The pleasures of being in love are enhanced tenfold by the benefits of regular Power Yoga practice. Power Yoga turns sex into a heightened spiritual experience in these ways:

- ✔ **Physically:** Yoga benefits your sexual performance by aiding the functions of your circulatory system, glands, and nerves. And regularly practicing Power Yoga postures and routines gives you more flexibility, muscle tone, and endurance.

- ✔ **Mentally:** Power Yoga can make you a lovemaking powerhouse. It frees your mind from stress, so you're more relaxed and compassionate. Power Yoga can also help you to channel the flow of your natural "electricity," or *prana* energy, through your body as well as the body of the lover you embrace. You'll notice the pure quality of your happiness, joy, and love. You'll also feel the integrity of your touch, a touch that comes from within and transcends the skin to touch your very soul and the soul of your lover. Your lovemaking will vibrate with the passionate, rhythmic waves of energy produced by your relaxed and powerful body.

Power Yoga is a turn-on, in every aspect of the word.

Part II
Preparing to Practice

The 5th Wave By Rich Tennant

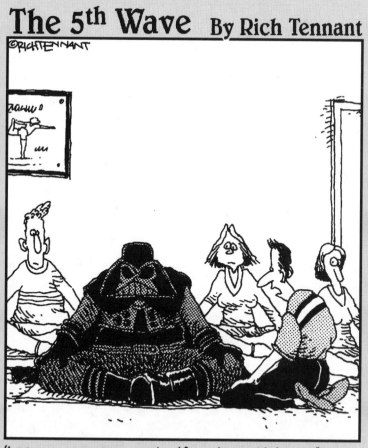

"Okay, you've got the breathing down, but wouldn't you be more comfortable in a different workout suit?"

In this part . . .

What kind of equipment do you need to practice Power Yoga? Not much: a mat, maybe a wall — a blanket, a pillow or two, a strap if you want some props. Where can you practice? Almost anywhere: in your home, in a studio, in your backyard — especially in your backyard or anyplace outdoors (you get bonus points!). When should you practice? Sunrise and sunset are especially good times to tap into the energy of the universe, but you can set your practice time to suit your schedule. How do you find a teacher? Ask your friends, look in the phone book, surf the Internet. The chapters in this part give you in-depth answers to the practical questions.

Chapter 4

Embracing Power Yoga Everyday

To adopt a Power Yoga lifestyle, you don't have to work out all day; believe me, that wouldn't be relaxing at all! Instead, you simply need to recognize Power Yoga as being more than a physical practice — think of it as a way of life and a state of mind. Power Yoga is a good fitness program because it teaches you the art of channeling your body's energy and its disciplined practices toward whatever path you choose in life. When you look beyond fitness to conceptualize the goal of Power Yoga as *empowerment*, you can use the practice to live life on your own terms, as your own person.

The Power Yoga lifestyle stretches more than your muscles; it often opens you up to a respect for nature, an interest in health, and an appreciation for your body. In the Power Yoga lifestyle, you apply the concepts of yogic thought and philosophy to the way you see your world, the way you interact with others, the decisions you make, and the food you eat.

This chapter takes a close look at both the practical and the beyond-the-mat aspects of Power Yoga. If you're considering "full-power" Power Yoga, this chapter is for you!

Planning a Powerful Practice

Power Yoga isn't about desperate competition or pushing yourself to work harder, faster, or better than everyone else. Competition can be a good thing, but it serves no purpose here. Power Yoga is about self-improvement through self-knowledge. By being in touch with your mind and body, you use Power

Yoga to achieve a balance between strength and softness, between physical exertion and mental relaxation.

Don't get me wrong; as you practice Power Yoga, you find that you become better able to assume and hold postures, and your "toolkit" of exercises and routines continually expands. But even as you become stronger and more accomplished in your practice, you should strive to achieve even greater focus and relaxation. Your workouts should become more challenging — not harder.

This list offers some good ideas for achieving the physical goals of your Power Yoga practice:

- ✔ Maintain a regular practice schedule
- ✔ Rotate practice routines
- ✔ Pace yourself
- ✔ Increase your workout time and intensity gradually
- ✔ Respect your limits of strength and flexibility
- ✔ Maintain a peaceful, relaxed approach
- ✔ Progress at your own pace

Change your routine from one week to the next so that you maintain a balanced program that includes strength, flexibility, and aerobic training. If you don't have enough time to finish your practice in one session, split up your routine over two or three days rather than try to cram too much into one session. Keep a peaceful, relaxed approach to your practice, and you'll progress quickly while maintaining your peace of mind. In Yoga, winners finish last!

And finally, set reasonable goals for your workout. You live in a world of extremes, but in Power Yoga, you're looking for balance. Pick a routine that's suited to your fitness level and personal goals, and then enjoy it. Don't burn all your fuel in the first few exercises of your routine; save enough energy to get to the end of the exercises. I don't like to sound like a dictator, but you definitely should *not* do these things in the course of your Power Yoga practice:

- ✔ Don't pick a routine beyond your comfort or skill level.
- ✔ Don't use up all your energy before you get half the way through your routine.
- ✔ Don't try to compete with others in your class.
- ✔ Don't neglect your relaxation time.
- ✔ Don't ignore pain and push yourself to the limit.

In other words, go with the flow!

Finding a Place for Your Practice

Your individual circumstances and preference determine where you choose to practice Power Yoga. You may have a perfect (or at least darned good) spot in your home, or you may prefer to practice in a Yoga studio. And the chances are good that you'll choose different locations at different times, to suit your energy and mood on any particular day. But whatever environment you choose, you need to be sure it offers a few basic features to make your Power Yoga practice safe, effective, and enjoyable. In this section, I talk about some of those features so you can choose a great Yoga workout location in your home, outdoors, or in a professional studio.

Making space in your place

To make Power Yoga a part of your life, you need a space in your home to practice. Make sure that space has these qualities:

- ✔ A couple of feet of solid wall to use during wall postures.
- ✔ A sturdy chair, a pillow, a Yoga practice mat and any blocks, straps, or other Yoga props you choose.
- ✔ Warmth, cleanliness, and quiet.
- ✔ Windows, so you can enjoy natural light and plenty of fresh air.

Make the room as pleasant and comfortable as you can — consider decorating the room with an eye toward creating a spiritual retreat, with tranquil lighting, soft music, and colors and textures that have a calming effect on you. And don't forget to add some plants to your Yoga space. The plants give you plenty of clean air and keep you more connected to other living things, even when you practice alone.

You may even want to create a sacred space. I have a little room with an altar in my house. An altar is just a space, like a little table or a mantle, that has things on and around it that remind you of your spirituality and your connection to the earth. Mine has candles, some rocks and stones I have collected from my journeys, and pictures that mean a lot to me. You can decorate yours with anything that connects you to your spiritual self.

Going to someone else's space

If you choose to practice in a Yoga studio, you have the help and support of an experienced teacher during your Power Yoga workout. This expert assistance comes in handy, especially when you're a beginner. Working out in a studio also gives you the benefit of group energy and socialization during your Power Yoga practice, so even experienced yogis and yoginis participate in studio classes.

Sometimes the best plan is to practice Power Yoga in the studio a few times each week, and use what you learn there in your at-home practice on the other days. Choose a studio and teacher you feel comfortable with, and don't hesitate to practice with different teachers occasionally. You can discover something new from every Power Yoga practitioner you work with, so don't limit your knowledge by limiting your Power Yoga experiences.

I give you the nitty-gritty on finding a teacher in Chapter 6.

Practicing in the great outdoors

Practicing Power Yoga in nature helps you feel more connected to the earth and makes it easier to tap into *prana,* your vital life-force energy.

If you have a quiet, isolated outdoor location where you can practice Power Yoga during good weather, you're all set! If your outdoor space is less tranquil, don't give up. As you become more familiar with Power Yoga techniques of concentration, you get better at blocking out the distractions of your environment and focusing on the benefits of fresh air, sunshine, and contact with the earth.

But don't let bad weather or a lack of outdoor space separate you from nature. After any practice, you can take a short walk, look up at the clouds, and breathe in the fresh air. The relaxed state that your practice puts you in helps you to more fully appreciate the beauty of nature.

Setting Aside the Time

I know that making time for your Power Yoga practice is hard sometimes; heck, sometimes it's hard for me. You probably have a busy, stressful life. In fact, you may have first decided to try Power Yoga to reduce some of that stress. But you have to make time to practice. Thinking about practicing doesn't help you nearly as much as *doing* it. I promise you this: The more you embrace the concepts and practices of Power Yoga in your life, the easier and more natural those practices become. And the more benefits they provide.

The irony is that when you make time for your practice, you're better able to focus on the real-life tasks at hand. You let go of the clutter in your mind, and you're able to think more clearly. When your Power Yoga practice becomes a Power Yoga lifestyle, you find that your workouts are a means of honing your problem-solving skills. And after standing on one foot for a while, you're better able to focus on whatever needs your attention!

Try to practice at least twice every week and work up to four times a week. After practicing for three or four weeks, you can increase the length and intensity of your workout. If you get sore and tired, return to a shorter, easier routine and increase the length and intensity when your energy returns and your soreness eases. Always respect your own limits.

Your practice sessions should last at least 30 minutes — an hour is better. Sunset and sunrise are the most powerful practice times, because they tend to be the most tranquil periods of the day. But any time is good for Power Yoga, so choose a schedule that works for you. And that schedule should include days off, too. I don't recommend that you practice Power Yoga every day of the week — occasional days of rest only increase the powerful effect of your practice. See Table 4-2 for my idea of a good practice schedule.

Many people find that regularly working out at the same time of day gives them the most benefit from their practice. Maintaining a consistent practice time gives you a better barometer for gauging your progress. You're at the same place in your day's activities and your energy and mood are at the same point in their daily cycle; as a result, you can better judge the effect of your practice.

Some powerfully good advice

As you prepare to launch into your first full Power Yoga routine, I have some words of wisdom that may make *all* your Power Yoga workouts easier:

- **Cross-train with other activities:** You'll progress faster if you incorporate other physical activity into your weekly schedule along with your Power Yoga. Try fast walking, light bike riding, swimming, or any other activity that you enjoy. If possible, you should do at least three 15-minute sessions of other physical activities every week. Approach these activities with the same yogic attitude that you apply to your Power Yoga workouts.

- **Watch your diet and nutrition:** To really put the power in your Power Yoga, consider making a moderate nutritional improvement by following a lower-fat and higher-fiber diet. Power Yoga builds your awareness of your physical condition, and it may inspire you to take positive actions in other areas of your life. (I talk more about Power Yoga and nutrition in Chapter 22.)

- **Boost your karma:** Don't let the good feeling you build during your Power Yoga routine go to waste; spread the good stuff around by giving someone a compliment, phoning a friend, or spending extra time with your family. Everything you do to build your feeling of inner peace benefits your Power Yoga practice. (The reverse is true, as well; Power Yoga practice makes it easier to feel calm and peaceful in stressful situations.)

Preparing Your Body

If you want to be a basketball player, you need to be tall; for football, your perfect body is strong, large, and fast. Dancers dream of bodies with perfect grace, balance, and rhythm. But what about yogis and yoginis? What's the perfect body for practicing Power Yoga? Congratulations, it's *yours!* That's right; every body — short, tall, old, young, fast, slow, thick, thin, graceful, not-so-graceful — is perfect for practicing Yoga. And, the more you practice, the "perfecter" you get. That's a good deal, isn't it?

Your body shape, bone structure, height, and weight are unique, and so are your physical and mental objectives. And every Power Yoga routine is unique, too, in the way its exercises are structured and sequenced to help certain body types strive toward specific fitness goals. If you just run out and start working through the first Power Yoga routine you meet, you may find it difficult, uncomfortable, and darned unappealing. Like anything else, you need to attend to first things first. Check out your current fitness level, so you know just where you stand on the road to fitness. Then choose the Power Yoga routine that takes you from ground zero to your fitness goal.

In this section, I walk you through a pre-routine checkup and throw in some extra tips to help you glide through your first Power Yoga session, like a butterfly on a springtime breeze. I show you how to prepare your mind and body for a positive experience in Power Yoga and how to set reasonable goals for your practice. I even provide a chart that can help you blend your Power Yoga routines with your other favorite fitness activities, to create a customized and complete fitness program.

Evaluating your current fitness level

Power Yoga is a balanced approach to fitness that encompasses strength, flexibility, and *aerobic* conditioning. (*Aerobic* exercise improves respiratory and circulatory functions. In order for an exercise to be aerobic, you must sustain continuous movement for at least 3 to 5 minutes.) No matter how active or inactive your lifestyle is, your fitness plan needs to take these three fitness factors into account. Many of my students, for example, come to me in really great aerobic condition, because they run or participate in other active sports. But those same students may have neglected flexibility and strength training. I've found that this kind of fitness imbalance can lead to stress, fatigue, and sports-related injuries.

Don't worry — this fitness evaluation isn't a test you pass or fail. Its purpose is strictly to help you evaluate your fitness "balance" and choose which Power Yoga routines are best for you.

In Table 4-1, I ask you to rate your aerobic condition, strength, flexibility, endurance, balance, and coordination on a scale where 4 means excellent,

3 is good, 2 is average and 1 is poor. Use the samples in the following list to guide you.

- ✔ **Aerobic condition:** If you get out of breath walking out to your car, give yourself a 1. If you jog or participate in sports on a regular basis, chalk up a 4.

- ✔ **Balance and coordination:** If you have a tendency to stumble and fall, and have trouble catching a ball or tossing something at a target, give yourself a low score here. But if you can hit the recycling bin from across the room, you're an ace bicyclist, or can walk across a narrow log spanning a creek or river, you get a 4 in this category.

- ✔ **Endurance:** If you can't do an aerobic activity for more than a few minutes without getting worn out, give yourself a 1 in this category. If you can bicycle, swim, jog, or perform other aerobic activities for hours, rate your endurance at 4.

- ✔ **Energy:** If you tend to hit the couch between dinner and bedtime, have a hard time getting up in the morning, and rarely feel like working out or performing any physical activity, your energy levels are low. If you regularly participate in some physical activity, and can happily pass up that evening lounge time for something more physically challenging, give yourself a 3 or 4.

- ✔ **Flexibility:** If you groan when you stoop or stand and suffer regular muscle and joint stiffness, your flexibility ranks as a 1 or 2; if you regularly bend, stoop, twist, lift, and stretch without pain or discomfort, you're a 3 or 4 in this category.

- ✔ **Strength:** If you live a very non-physical life and rarely if ever exert or work your muscles, give yourself a 1 in this category; if you work your muscles on a regular basis, give yourself a 3 or 4.

I also ask you questions about your experience with Yoga. Remember, Power Yoga is about self-improvement, not competition! If you're honest with yourself, this evaluation can help you find an appropriate exercise routine. If you've never tried Yoga before, give yourself 1 point in this category. Six month's Yoga experience gets you 2 points, a year equals 3 points; and two or more years gives you 4 points.

Table 4-1	Personal Fitness Evaluation
Fitness Area	*Your Score*
Aerobic condition	
Balance and coordination	
Endurance	

(continued)

Table 4-1 *(continued)*	
Fitness Area	*Your Score*
Energy	
Flexibility	
Strength	
Abdominal muscles	
Legs	
Arms	
Involvement in Yoga	

Add up all the points that you assigned yourself in the evaluation. The result tells you your fitness level, based on the following guidelines:

9 to 14 points = Level 1/Beginner

15 to 21 points = Level 2/Intermediate I

22 to 29 points = Level 3/Intermediate II

30 points or more = Level 4/Advanced

Checking in with the doc

Before you start a Power Yoga practice at any level, give your doctor a buzz to get medical approval for your plan. If you think your M.D. may not be familiar with Power Yoga, take this book with you to your appointment.

I'm not a doctor — and I don't even play one on TV — but I do know a few red flags that may signal the need for caution in proceeding down the road to Power Yoga. For example, you should avoid inverted Yoga poses if you have any of these health problems:

✔ **Floating or detached retina:** This is a condition in which the retina of the eye is detached and floating. It usually results from injury to the eye.

✔ **Very high blood pressure:** Ask your doctor if your blood pressure is significantly high and whether he or she thinks you should avoid inverted postures.

✔ **During menstruation:** You're cleansing the body during menstruation, and inverted poses may hinder the natural elimination of toxins. This is a personal choice; some women find that inverted poses don't bother them at all during menstruation.

Can't cha hear me talkin' to ya?

Many times, when I'm teaching a Yoga workshop, someone will limp up to me, wincing in pain, and say, "How can I do this Lotus Pose when my knee hurts so much that I can't cross my legs?" Well, my answer to that question is very simple: don't do *anything* that causes you pain. And certainly don't keep doing something that's been causing you pain over a period of time. Wise up and listen to your body. If your body feels pain when you assume a posture, don't do it. Shed your ego, and stay away from that pose for a while. Chances are good that if you give your body a chance to catch up or to heal from an injury, you eventually will be able to assume the posture without pain. That's the whole idea of Power Yoga — gain *without* pain.

If you have any questions about your physical ability to practice Power Yoga, check with your doctor. If you begin Power Yoga practice with a Yoga instructor, that instructor will probably ask you about any existing medical conditions and whether you've talked to your doctor about practicing Power Yoga. Make sure to notify your Yoga teacher about any injuries you've experienced or any blood sugar problems you have. And tell your teacher about the fitness level that you assigned to yourself in the evaluation table in this chapter. Remember, this is the time for full disclosure! Your Yoga instructor can work with you effectively only if you lay all your cards on the table.

Definitely disclose any history of surgery within the last year, any chronic disease, and any diagnosed back problems or back surgeries.

Avoiding (Ouch!) injuries

Avoiding injuries is much easier than overcoming them. When you feel pain in your muscles or joints, your body is sending you a clear signal: "Hey, I'm talking to you. Are you listening? That hurts worse than the time you dropped a hammer on my toe. So give me a break, and stop it!" Don't forget that your body and your mind are partners in Power Yoga. You aren't fighting your body to "make" it get better; you're helping it become better. Give your body the respect it deserves; listen to it and follow its wishes. That's the surest way to avoid injuries.

In the spirit of the good adviser, I give you my favorite list of safety first ideas for practicing Power Yoga:

- ✔ Practice in a warm environment (even though you should have fresh air coming in, if possible).
- ✔ Enter and exit postures very gracefully and cautiously. You're respecting your body, not making it conform.

✔ Move softly and fluidly between poses.

✔ Use counter-stretches. If you do a series of forward bends and then a series of backward bends, stretch on one side and then stretch on the other.

✔ Don't practice every day. Take some days off (sometimes, even a number of days in a row) to let your body relax from the workout.

Think of your body as a wonderful machine, with lots of working parts run by the ultimate computer: *your mind*. If you take care of yourself, eat right, practice Power Yoga, and get plenty of rest, you'll have a sweet-running machine.

Getting Your Head Ready for the Trip

After you check your fitness level, it's time to explore a bit more about the physical nature of the Power Yoga exercises and how to get the most out of them, so that you're better able to plan routines that fit your goals and lifestyle.

A bit of "head prep" can help you psych up for the most powerful Power Yoga workouts (and their results). So check through this pre-practice list, and then I'll leave you with a Power Yoga exercise to help you glide into the next phase of the journey. Use these ideas to keep your mental approach to Power Yoga on track:

✔ Keep a calm, relaxed mind throughout your exercise.

✔ Embrace practice with a positive mental attitude.

✔ Enjoy your practice; make it fun!

✔ Get plenty of rest and relaxation.

As you move into more challenging exercises, keep your mind relaxed and focused. If your mind starts to struggle with the work, your body will struggle, too. Keep it light, keep it loose, and don't sweat it. Before you start each Power Yoga routine, take a few moments to focus your mind on positive thoughts and visualize yourself completing a great session.

Above all, keep your sense of humor; laughter really *is* the best medicine — in Power Yoga and in life. Laughter can help you avoid injuries, enjoy your practice more, and remain in general good health. And if you start to feel a drop in your enthusiasm, vary your routine, change your schedule a bit, or try some partner Power Yoga exercises.

Power Yoga is a great thing you're doing for *you*. Listen to your body and your head, and you'll find the right path to your ultimate Power Yoga destination.

Plugging into positive energy

Want to be really powerful? You will be when your Power Yoga practice teaches you to be soft. If that sounds contradictory, just think for a moment about water. Water is one of the softest elements of our planet, and yet it can carve through mountains and move huge boulders. Water's greatest strength lies in its persistent flow. The Power Yoga lifestyle encourages you to develop the same soft and subtle strength in dealing with your daily challenges.

Power Yoga generates an enormous amount of positive energy, both mental and physical. As you adopt a Power Yoga lifestyle, you find that you can use this energy in everything you do.

As you become more practiced in Power Yoga, you'll find that you're increasingly aware of the energy you generate and the energy of those around you. Living a Power Yoga lifestyle encourages you to appreciate the strength of softness, the power of living in the moment, the force of patience, and the revitalizing benefits of seeing the world around you through your heart as well as through your eyes. Your Power Yoga routines build your physical energy, but a Power Yoga lifestyle puts you in touch with the energy of everything around you.

Harnessing your emotions

If you lose your cool and fly out of control, you demonstrate weakness, not strength. You can't function at your best when your emotions take over. You don't think clearly, and you make bad decisions. From your firm, grounded position as a Power Yoga practitioner, you can deal with any situation by projecting calm, tranquil strength. When you tap into the strength of a Power Yoga lifestyle, you keep it light, keep it loose, and never let them see you sweat.

If you find yourself tensing up, use your yoga breathing techniques to calm down and find your center. Take slow, deep inhalations, and exhale slowly and completely. Tense and relax your muscles to help unknot them, and (if possible) close your eyes for a few moments and visualize your body relaxing. As you let go of the tension you'll feel more alert and better able to respond to the situation at hand.

Clearing the cobwebs

You can use Power Yoga to get yourself right when things just feel wrong. If you use Power Yoga when you're feeling unproductive, for example, a miracle happens! Seemingly insurmountable tasks are possible, and you know exactly where to begin. If you're a student studying for exams, you find that you can recharge with Power Yoga. You can jump up and strike a pose whenever you find yourself getting distracted during your studies.

This yogic moment

A Yoga master drove up to the drive-through window of a fast food burger shack. The place didn't get many Yoga masters, and the employees couldn't wait to hear what this odd vegetarian would order. The drive-through attendant said, "May I take your order?" The Yoga master replied," Just a moment, please." The attendant waited a few minutes, as cars backed up behind the Yoga master, and still no order came through the speaker. The attendant asked again, "What is it that you would like to have?" The Yoga master again said, "Just a moment is all I need."

The Power Yoga lifestyle keeps you young — you're physically fit and mentally sharp. Whether you're playing a game of golf or chasing your kids around the yard, when Power Yoga is part of your life, you have an edge. Power Yoga helps you rise above the competition, even when your opponent is the aging process!

Blending Power Yoga with Other Fitness Activities

Power Yoga complements — and is complemented by — other physical activities. If you're interested in boosting the benefits of your Power Yoga workouts, you can use the chart in this section to create a customized, blended physical workout routine.

The following table is just a general guide giving you my suggestions for a blended workout week that balances other activities with Power Yoga routines. Remember that Power Yoga is a complete fitness routine in and of itself. As you become fit, however, and you have more energy for more activities, you can use these suggestions as a launching pad for expanding your fitness program.

Table 4-2 is a sample week long fitness program. The activities work to build all the areas of balanced fitness — aerobics, endurance, flexibility, and balance. I also allow plenty of time for rest. Under each day of the week, the chart recommends times (in minutes) for specific activities. (The minimum time is my recommendation for Level 1 students; and the maximum is for Level 4 students; Level 2 and Level 3 students should choose times between these parameters.) Choose strength and flexibility routines from the strength-training and flexibility training chapters of this book.

Don't forget the R&R!

When you're planning your Power Yoga practice and deciding which exercises and routines are right for you, don't forget to add the critical ingredients of *rest* and *relaxation* to your plan. I've mentioned the importance of nourishment for your body. As you make more demands of your muscles, joints, and tendons, you need to be sure that you're giving them the fuel to meet those demands. But your body can't live on food alone; it needs rest to recharge its batteries. During your hectic days, don't forget to take a deep breath and enjoy the moment periodically. And get plenty of sleep and quality relaxation time *every day*. If you keep your body well rested *and* well exercised, you get twice the benefit from your Power Yoga practice — in half the time.

Table 4-2	A Balanced Weekly Fitness Plan						
Activity	*Mon.*	*Tues.*	*Wed.*	*Thur.*	*Fri.*	*Sat.*	*Sun.*
Walk or jog			20–60		30–90		off
Bicycle		20–90		20–90			off
Other aerobic	20–60						off
Power Yoga (flexibility)		30–60				30–60	off
Power Yoga (strength)				30–60			off
Swimming		20–45					off
Weight lifting	20–60		20–60				off
Hiking						45–90	off

Just relax all day Sunday or any other day of your choice.

Every fitness program is an individualized pursuit, so you need to create one that you like and that works well for you. Just remember to avoid the competitive urge and respect your own limits.

I live in the mountainous area of South Lake Tahoe, California, and you can believe there are a lot of athletes around here. And everybody's into something different — bicycling, rock-climbing, skiing, and so on. But almost everyone tends to specialize in the activity they're best at, so they look good while they're working out. All the really good athletes, though, know they can't limit their exercise to just one type. Cross-training — incorporating a number of different types of exercise into your regular program — is the only way to stay fit and at the top of your game.

Power Yoga is an aerobic exercise in and of itself; but you can see significant gains in your endurance if you add other types of aerobic activities such as handball, jogging, bicycling, and so on to your program. Aerobic activity improves the strength of your lungs and cardiovascular system.

Chapter 5

Getting the Skinny on Yoga Gear

· ·

In This Chapter

▶ Dressing up Yoga style

▶ Shopping (without dropping) for basic gear

▶ Propping up your Yoga practice

· ·

You can most certainly practice Yoga without any special gear or clothing — all you really need is a quiet mind, your birthday suit, that smile on your face, and a piece of ground to practice on.

But I don't live under a rock, you know. I know that in the twenty-first century, people start any fitness or recreation program with a shopping trip. So have a little fun with your Power Yoga adventure, and get some gear! In Yoga, *gear* means "clothing" to make you feel better and "props" to make your workout easier and more productive.

In this chapter, you find out how to get all dressed up when you have a Yoga place to go. Your choice of Yoga clothing makes your Power Yoga more enjoyable, creative, and comfortable; I can show you how to find the fashions that best fit your body *and* your mind when you're doing Power Yoga.

I give you the lowdown on props, too — whether you're looking for the ancient, straight-from-nature variety or the latest in high-tech Yogic gizmos. I tell you what does what, what's hot, what's not, what to buy, and where to buy it. So what are you waiting for? Put on your shoes, grab your wallet, and let's go shopping!

Looking Good! Fashion and Yoga

What to wear to Power Yoga class? You surely don't want to arrive late, wearing dirty mud boots and skintight bluejeans. That get-up won't cut it, not even in California.

You may not have spent much time in a Yoga studio, so how can you find out what everyone wears in the Power Yoga world? Well, you read this chapter. I give you a little peek through the window of a studio during a typical Power Yoga workout (figuratively, of course — remember, Power Yoga success requires a healthy imagination). That way, you can see for yourself what's fashionable in Power Yoga today.

You've heard the expression "no boundaries," haven't you? Well, it certainly applies to Yoga threads. You can wear anything that's comfortable, as long as it doesn't restrict your movement. You're going to bend, twist, and fold your body in a variety of shapes, and your clothing needs to go with you.

Some people wear layers, beginning their workout with a heavy top and sweatpants over their leotards or shorts and then stripping down as they warm up. As you become familiar with your body's response to your Power Yoga routines, you'll find the clothing weight and type that's best for you.

You may work up quite a sweat during your Power Yoga session. Always be sure to bring some sort of light coverup to prevent getting chilled as you leave the studio. If it's cold outside, plan to spend some time cooling down before you walk out the door.

Keep in mind, too, that every studio maintains its own climate, and the studio's temperature of choice may be too hot or cold for your tastes. That's why it's really important that you take plenty of options (clothing layers) with you to your first session, so you can be comfortable, no matter what the studio's thermostat says. (Most studios have locker rooms or changing facilities where you can switch togs, if necessary.)

Becoming a fashionable yogini

Cool! There's a session in progress now. And look at some of those women! They're dressed to the max, wearing color-coordinated leotards or tight-fitting shorts, matching tops, and headbands. Lots of women prefer to wear cotton-based leotards with a bit of stretch, especially nice organic cotton duds, and others are wearing high-tech Lycra workout clothes that wick away sweat while they stretch every which way.

Preparing for the cool-down

Power Yoga creates heat, and as your workout progresses, you can expect to sweat. That's great, because it means your body heat is up, your heart and lungs are working, and your circulatory and respiratory systems are getting a good run, too. But when the power drops at the end of the session, you're going to be left a bit damp and flushed. Most Power Yoga sessions end with a relaxation exercise, and it can be pretty hard to relax when you're shivering and cold! I recommend that you bring a blanket to cover up with during the relaxation phase of your workout. In fact, ask your teacher if the studio keeps blankets on hand for just this very purpose. Lots of people throw on socks and a sweatshirt for relaxation, especially in the winter.

But notice, too, that lots of these women are wearing sweat pants, pajama bottoms, loose cotton shorts, oversized T-shirts, and simple cotton tank tops. In other words, the fashion word for women doing Power Yoga seems to be "choice." You can wear any clothing that gives you plenty of unrestricted movement and, most importantly, is comfortable.

Don't forget the support! Some women seem comfortable and get adequate breast support by wearing tight-fitting stretch tops, while others wear sports bras to cut down on the "bounce" and give their breasts the support they need. Power Yoga is an active endeavor, so dress accordingly. Find a bra or tank top that doesn't move around much so you stay covered no matter what position you move into.

Yogis need fashion, too

And what about the guys? Men in the Power Yoga studio are dressed just as diversely as women are. Some wear tight-fitting workout shorts or long leotards. Others wear loose-fitting sweat pants, pajama bottoms, shorts, T-shirts, or tank tops. Some of the guys are shirtless, while others are sporting layers. And, of course, a few of them wear headbands and wristbands.

Like the women in the class, men tend to choose clothing that's comfortable and in keeping with their usual clothing preferences.

Casual observation doesn't tell you much about the underwear these dudes are sporting, but I can tell you it's strictly a matter of personal choice. You don't really need a jock strap when you're doing Power Yoga, though some guys choose to wear them. You don't have to worry about getting kicked or knocked down in Power Yoga, so groin injuries aren't a factor, as they are in contact sports. Personally, I find jock straps to be uncomfortable during practice, and I just rely on 100 percent cotton underwear. The ancient yogis didn't bother with any kind of "masculine" support, so as I said, your Power Yoga underwear (or lack thereof) is strictly a matter of personal comfort.

Shopping for Power Yoga Gear

You can dress up or down for your Power Yoga sessions — let your fashion conscience be your guide! If you need to stock up on some hot Yoga fashion numbers, you shouldn't have much trouble finding a nearby source of workout clothing. In fact, your sources are limited only by the amount of money you're willing to spend.

You can choose from many types of workout clothing and athletic apparel for your Power Yoga practice. With the popularity of exercise today, you can find workout clothing in department stores, athletic stores, and even thrift shops. Lots of online and mail-order sources for Yoga clothing and gear are waiting on your business, too; just pick up a copy of a Yoga magazine or go online and search for "Yoga apparel" or "Yoga gear" using your favorite search engine.

Of course, I have my favorite sources for Yoga clothing and props, which I list in Appendix B, at the end of this book.

To Prop or Not to Prop?

To prop or not to prop? Yeah — that's the question! Do you think that you can suffer the slings and arrows of Power Yoga without special props, or do you feel destined to become spiritually connected with some fun, comfortable Power Yoga gear? Okay, I'll leave Shakespeare alone for a minute so you can take a look what props are, what they're good for, and the pros and cons of using them in Power Yoga.

Props are pads, blocks, mats, straps, pillows, blankets, and other objects that may be helpful for beginning yogis. When you first attempt certain Power Yoga postures, you may have trouble keeping your balance, or assuming or maintaining certain positions comfortably. With a pillow here or a block there, what had been a wobbly, unsatisfying perch becomes a comfortable, secure pose. Some people swear by props; others avoid them like the plague.

Go ahead and be a nature boy (or girl)

You don't have to use any props to have a great Power Yoga experience. Even if you decide to go with some blocks, straps, or pillows, you should occasionally try your practice without any props. (I do recommend, however, that you use a purchased Yoga mat or a soft, grassy spot outdoors.) Don't get into a rut with your practice. By flying solo (without props) occasionally, you can have a rejuvenating Power Yoga experience that reminds you of why you were using props in the first place. And it may convince you that you don't need them anymore.

Props can very often assist you in your practice, especially if you're feeling awkward, inflexible, and unstable with a posture. Yoga props can be a great help in getting you started and making you comfortable with Power Yoga postures and exercises. Other props, like eye pillows, simply make you feel more comfortable. Many students like to cover their eyes with eye pillows during relaxation poses. Some students like to relax with blankets under their knees or neck pillows under their necks.

Of course, you don't *have* to use props. As a matter of fact, props were discouraged by many of the original teachers of Power Yoga. For the first ten years or so of my practice, I refused to use any props. I thought they were unnatural, unnecessary distractions that really diminished the purity and focus of Yoga. Since then, I've come to realize that Yoga props can help people get started and successfully expand their Power Yoga routines. That said, I still think that everyone should strive to use minimal props in Power Yoga. After you get your moves in the groove, you should be able to kiss most aids good-bye and fly solo through your Power Yoga routines. When you're practicing Power Yoga, you want to flow smoothly from pose to pose. That kind of smooth transition isn't easy when you're shuffling around blocks and straps.

On the other hand, you may not need any props at all. If you're in great shape, have some experience in Yoga, and already enjoy pretty good balance, strength, and flexibility, you probably can get through most Power Yoga routines comfortably without props. (You probably want to continue using a mat, however.)

I suggest that you try some of the props available in your Yoga studio. See what works best for you and then do what feels natural. If props help you get with the Power Yoga program, go for it! Periodically, you can try the postures without props; if you discover that you don't need them anymore, you can toss the props aside. It's a fluid process, and you're in control.

Before you can decide whether or not you want to use Yoga props, you need to know more about what they are and what they'll do. In the following sections, I explain some of the most commonly used Yoga props and how to use them.

Taking a magic carpet ride

If I were going to say that you really need any Yoga prop, I would recommend a good mat. For at least 10 years, I practiced Yoga daily with my brother David and a few close friends. During all that time, we rarely used any Yoga props at all — with the exception of cotton mats. We used those mats daily for years, and they made our practice more comfortable, safer, and more enjoyable.

In fact, I might say that the true path to enlightenment is a nice, light, soul-levitating mat. I recommend that you use a good mat when you practice Yoga. One especially made for Yoga, too. The mat makes your practice more comfortable and more stable. It also gives you a warm pad for relaxation exercises and a "home base" to work from in class.

You can choose from a variety of Yoga mat styles and types:

✔ **Cotton mat (a classic):** Beautiful, 100 percent cotton mats are wonderful for Power Yoga workouts. They feel good on your skin, and green cotton mats (made from cotton grown without pesticides and processed without bleach and harmful dyes) are good for the environment, too. You can get cotton mats that are thick and stuffed, but these are better used for relaxation and restorative Yoga. For Power Yoga, stick with a cotton rug-like mat.

✔ **Rubber mat:** Sticky rubber mats help keep your feet and hands from sliding out from under you when you assume postures. These mats give you much better traction than do cotton mats, yet they have a somewhat unnatural feel, and their manufacturing processes aren't always environmentally friendly. These days, you can choose from many different styles, textures, and thickness. Check out different ones and see what works best for you.

Almost all sticky mats are a little less than sticky — in fact, they're downright slippery — when new. You have to break them in, so get moving!

✔ **Combination (best of both worlds):** I recommend that you use both types of mats; you can keep the rubber mat on the bottom and the cotton mat on top; flip them over to get the foundation you need. Use the sticky mat when you need extra traction and the cotton mat when you want to rest on a natural-feeling surface during a posture.

✔ **Computerized mat:** The mat of the future will be computerized to take you automatically through the Yoga poses while you think about what's for dinner. (Don't hold your breath waiting for this one!)

As with most Power Yoga decisions, only you can determine what type of mat is best for you. I recommend that beginners seriously consider using the two-mat combo. Most types of mats can be purchased through magazines such as *Yoga International* and *Yoga Journal,* or you may be able to buy one at your local Yoga studio. A local studio probably will let you try out various types of mats so you can pick out one that works perfectly for you. You may even find cotton mats in import stores or department stores. (You can find plenty of sources for Yoga mats in Appendix B, as well as subscription information for the magazines I mention.)

Strapping up your Power Yoga workout

Straps in Power Yoga practice have become as common as automobile seat belts. Straps can help you work out in many ways. They help you extend the reach of your hands, give you a handle to hold onto while balancing in poses, and can assist in supplying counter-tension during spinal twists and other postures. Yoga straps are usually 1-inch-wide strips of cotton or some cotton-blend fabric, and they come in a variety of lengths. Most straps are plain, although some have buckles.

The straps don't come with instructions, so you need to use your imagination a bit when deciding how straps work best in your Power Yoga practice. But if you're a beginner or if you have a body type that doesn't mold to the Yoga postures right away, straps can help you get the benefit of these postures even before you're able to conform your body to them on your own.

For example, if flexibility isn't your best physical trait, you may have difficulty reaching your toes in the Seated Forward Bend. Even if your toes seem a mile away, the strap can help you benefit from this posture. To use a strap with this pose, place it just below the balls of your feet and hold the ends in your hands. You get the stretching benefit to the back of the legs, even though you aren't yet able to get into the "official" pose. (***Remember:*** That benefit cannot occur when you round your back and hunch your shoulders.) Your feet remain straight, your calves get a good stretch, and you're on your way to becoming flexible enough to do the posture without aids!

Your teacher may use straps to help you get into the proper alignment for Power Yoga postures, too. For example, your teacher (or partner) may wrap a strap around your thighs and pull the strap ends to help you move deeper into your Downward Facing Dog pose (see the Cheat Sheet).

You can buy Yoga straps from any of the other Yoga prop sources mentioned in this chapter (and listed in Appendix B), but you don't have to get so fancy. I've seen people do just fine using old socks, towels, or cotton belts as straps in Power Yoga workouts. The choice is yours.

Playing with blocks

Now don't go stealing your children's building blocks; Yoga blocks are a bit different. Blocks are square supports made of wood, plastic, or foam, and they have many excellent uses in Power Yoga practice. Blocks are truly props, in that they can help prop you up into certain poses, such as raising your hips off the floor to help stretch your ankles and hips. Blocks also give you something to lean on during a standing or bending posture when your hand won't quite reach the mat. As you practice new postures and linking movements *(asanas and vinyasas),* you'll find other ways that blocks can help you achieve poses in comfort.

You can order blocks through Yoga magazines or your local Yoga studio. Then again, you can make your own out of a block of foam or wooden box. (If you make your own, be sure that any foam material is dense enough to provide adequate support and that wood blocks are sanded and smooth.) You can find sources for buying Yoga blocks in Appendix B, along with the other resources I list there.

Relaxing with flax eye pillows

Many students chose to use eye pillows during relaxation pose. Eye pillows are small pillows that you put on your eyes during your relaxation time at the end of your Power Yoga session. The gentle pressure helps your eyes relax and sink into your head.

The pillows are often made of rayon or silk or another smooth, silky fabric, which soothes the eyes. They are usually filled with flaxseeds that stay cool and have a soothing feel. Some are stuffed with lavender and other relaxing herbs, or have soothing herbs mixed with the flaxseed. You can also drip a few drops of essential lavender oil on your eye pillow to add to the relaxing sensation.

ALTERNATIVE

Discovering natural props

The popularity of Yoga has spawned an enormous variety of Yoga props and gear, most of which you can live without. In fact, back in the good old days (the late 1960s), I practiced Yoga outdoors about 75 percent of the time, using no prop other than a wise old oak tree (and it was more company than physical support). As my outdoor practice evolved, I discovered and began to use a number of natural props in my routines. So, you don't have to look to the catalogs for props — just look around outdoors. Here are some of my favorite natural props:

- **Rocks and tree stumps:** Rocks, logs, and tree stumps work just fine as natural blocks.

- **Tree vines and long grasses:** Vines (avoid the three-leaved, hairy vines of poison ivy, of course) and long grasses serve the same purpose as straps in a natural Power Yoga workout.

- **Leaves, moss, and grass:** Nature provides a number of good replacements for a Yoga workout mat. The feeling of working on a soft, natural grass mat is wonderful, but be aware that you have to contend with ants, ticks, and other undesirable elements on nature's turf.

- **Tree moss:** Tree moss makes a great eye pillow, providing complete darkness and a soothing touch during relaxation exercises. I've used soft tree moss this way on many occasions, but again, I've had to contend with bugs. You can compromise and buy some flaxseed eye pillows covered with green cotton or natural silk. These eye pillows are very soothing and 100 percent natural.

Simplicity is the road to happiness, and when you find yourself comfortably practicing Power Yoga in a natural atmosphere, it's the ultimate high! Practicing outdoors, using Mother Nature's homemade props, is a great way to experience the best possible Power Yoga workout.

Chapter 6

Finding a Yoga Teacher

After you get your Yoga books, videos, props, clothes, and maybe even an "I love Power Yoga" bumper sticker, you need to consider one other important aid in your quest to master Power Yoga — a good Power Yoga master. You don't really *need* a Power Yoga master, but you really can benefit from a good instructor. You can discover lots about Power Yoga from this book, and you can also find some good video and audiotapes to help you get started. But studying with a good teacher is definitely advantageous. A Power Yoga instructor can help you reach your full Power Yoga potential. Also, ongoing instruction can help you progress more quickly, be more comfortable with your power postures, avoid injuries, and enjoy your practice.

In this chapter, I show you what to look for in a Power Yoga instructor, how to find a good one, and what questions to ask. So grab your gear and head out to hunt down a guru!

Checking Out Teachers and Gurus

Happily, finding a good Yoga teacher is a bit easier today than it was during the time of the ancient Yoga masters. Even so, if you live in a small town or rural location, you may have to look around a bit to find a good Power Yoga instructor and studio. And you may need to test drive a few Power Yoga classes with one or two different instructors before you find the best fit. But the rewards of finding a first-class instructor are well worth the effort involved.

I'd walk a mile for a guru

The Sanskrit word *guru* means "teacher" (literally "weighty one" who dispels darkness). Until about 40 years ago, people who wanted to study Yoga had to travel great distances and endure many hardships on the quest for a good teacher. The lucky ones who survived the journey and actually located a Yoga teacher had to go through some extreme physical and mental tests to prove themselves worthy of being the Yoga guru's student. Today, Yoga is popular in all walks of life, and you don't have to trek up any mountains in your quest for an instructor. You may, however, have to look around a bit to find the teacher (or teachers) who work best with you. Each instructor is unique in his or her own way, so don't hesitate to play the field. As the song says, "You better shop around."

Don't get hung up on the idea of finding a guru rather than someone who simply goes by the title of teacher. Many ordinary Power Yoga teachers are disguised as gurus, and many gurus are disguised as ordinary teachers. The best instructors — regardless of title — are truthful, nonegotistical, compassionate, and friendly. Good Yoga instructors never stop their own learning process, and they never claim to have all the answers.

Before I actually studied with a guru, I envisioned the master Yoga teacher to be someone like Yoda from the movie *Star Wars*. I thought a guru had to be a person who lived in the woods, knew all things, led a perfect and ecologically balanced life, ate the perfect diet, was compassionate and understanding to all, and had no ego. I hate to shatter your dreams, but most of the popular gurus today can never fill Yoda's shoes (if he had worn any!).

You may never find all these qualities in a single Power Yoga instructor, and personally, I don't believe that you can find one perfect Power Yoga teacher who has all the answers. You have to look for the good in each instructor and then build your own guru within. By absorbing as much information as you can, you develop your own knowledge of Power Yoga, and that knowledge can help guide you toward further lessons. Some teachers have a great approach to teaching relaxation techniques, and others have the ability to always lead a class through the most powerful routines. You may find a class that's attended by someone you really want to partner with during Power Yoga, or you may discover an instructor who offers the best adjustments to your postures. That's all cool — variety is the spice of Power Yoga life. Life is a banquet, so why limit yourself to a single-serving learning experience?

Knowing what you're looking for

Before you actually go out looking for an instructor, you should first clarify what you seek. The following possibilities may help you define your dream Yoga experience:

- ✔ **Budget/monetary investment:** Regular, on-going group instruction usually runs anywhere from $5 to $25 a class, depending on what part of the country you're in and who's teaching the classes. For private instruction, expect to pay a minimum of $40 to $50 per hour; rates can go as high as $300 or more per hour, depending on the instructor's popularity.

- ✔ **Group or private instruction:** Group instruction usually takes place in a class setting with anywhere from 3 to 80 people or more. Group instruction offers the benefits of group incentive, energy, and social opportunities. The one-on-one approach of private instruction offers you much more personal attention and may help you discover more. You can even fine-tune your practice by combining the two, using individual instruction as a way of pinpointing challenges and solutions that you can then work on in your class.

- ✔ **Level of practice:** With the popularity of Yoga today, many teachers offer sessions at several levels — beginning to advanced. When you're scheduling a session with an instructor, be sure that you have some idea what level of instruction is right for you. If you have questions about your level, the instructor should be able to help you sort out the answers.

- ✔ **Time investment:** You can get by with as few as two or three 20-minute workouts a week, or you may choose to work out three hours a day, six days a week. You need to make sure that the instruction you want is available when you want it.

Asking all the right questions

After you locate a potential teacher, you need to ask the instructor some important questions. If you just walk into a class without finding out something about the instructor, his or her background, and his or her approach to Power Yoga, you may find yourself in a disappointing situation that you don't feel comfortable leaving.

Asking the instructor some questions up front is easier than walking out of a commitment to a full series of Power Yoga classes. Here are some good questions to ask any Power Yoga instructor whose class you're considering:

- ✔ **Can you tell me a bit about your background in Yoga including how long you've studied?** Try to find someone with a fair amount of experience, but don't judge the instructor's ability entirely on the answers to these questions. You're really just trying to get a sense of the length and quality of the person's background in Yoga and Power Yoga.

- ✔ **Are you certified with any organizations?** Yoga certification is a relatively new concept, yet it's available to teachers through a number of avenues. Again, if the instructor isn't certified, don't close the door in his or her face; lots of good teachers aren't certified. Still, this is helpful information for determining an instructor's training and background.

✔ **Can you accommodate my needs and level of practice?** It's always best to let the teacher know exactly what you're looking for. Are you hoping to heal specific injuries? Are you hoping to recover from insomnia? Do you want a challenging physical workout or a less vigorous stretching session? Make sure that any potential teacher can accommodate your goals.

✔ **Do you have any references?** If the teacher has been around awhile, he or she should be able to produce some local references.

And what do the answers to your questions tell you? The most experienced and popular teachers aren't always the best, and rookies aren't always the worst. Even when you know some things about an instructor's background, you still need to use your powers of personal assessment to line up the best instructor for your Power Yoga practice.

Being a good teacher has much to do with the qualities of the individual, such as communication, compassion, kindness, confidence, and sincerity. Look for these qualities in a Power Yoga instructor:

✔ **A calm, relaxed demeanor and a sharp, alert mind:** Ideally, you want to find an instructor who has some of the qualities that Power Yoga is known to provide to its practitioners — such as a calm, focused attitude and a sharp mind.

✔ **A patient approach to dealing with your questions:** If your teacher doesn't show an interest in your questions or doesn't take the time to answer them, you probably won't get the time and attention you need in class either.

✔ **A personality you feel comfortable with:** A person can be a great teacher, but if you don't feel comfortable with him or her, it's best to go elsewhere.

On the other hand, all Power Yoga instructors aren't necessarily going to have the right stuff. These traits should send you running from a potential instructor's class:

✔ **Certified by an unknown source in one weekend:** One of the downsides to the recent rush of Power Yoga popularity is that many certification-in-a-weekend sites have sprung up. Ask your potential instructor to tell you who conducted the certification program and how long the program lasted — beware if it was a quickie. (You can check out Appendix B for a partial list of instructors that I can vouch for.)

✔ **A high-pressure sales pitch:** Walk away from a teacher whose main concern is selling you a package deal. The instructor should listen to your goals and your interests in studying Power Yoga, instead of pressuring you to buy the "perfect package."

✔ **Little or no experience:** Instructors who have been practicing and teaching for less than a year have limited hands-on experience.

Looking Up, Down, and All Around

Power Yoga's popularity has soared in the last few years, and so have your avenues for finding a teacher. Depending on where you call home, you may have a variety of sources for Power Yoga instruction. Begin your quest in some of these places:

- **Health clubs:** Because of the popularity of Yoga and Power Yoga, you're likely to find classes offered at many of your local health clubs. Sometimes, the fee is included in your monthly dues.

- **High school and college classes:** Check your local high school and colleges; you may find that they offer some wonderful Power Yoga classes at reasonable prices.

- **Web sites:** You're living in the computer age, and the Internet offers a valuable path for finding Power Yoga instruction. Whether you're looking for a class, a workshop, or a teacher, you should try an online search for locating a source in your area.

- **Word of mouth:** Talk to people you know. With the popularity of Power Yoga today, you may know someone who is practicing Power Yoga or who knows of a studio or teacher in your area. Just remember that opinions about teachers are just like opinions about movies. You may well love a class that a friend didn't.

- **The Yellow Pages:** If you are looking for the best instruction in the most Yoga-conducive environment, a good Yoga studio is the way to go. The Yellow Pages of your local telephone directory is an excellent source to locate local studios and schools of Yoga. Look under Yoga, Fitness Instruction, and so on.

- **Yoga magazines:** If you're interested in Yoga workshops, teacher training, or retreats, Yoga magazines are the best source. Try *Yoga International* or *Yoga Journal.* (Other sources are listed in Appendix B of this book.)

Testing the Water before You Dive In

Before you sign up for a class, make sure that you meet and talk to the person who actually teaches the class, not just the owner of the studio. And if possible, try out a class or two before you commit to a full Power Yoga course. Some instructors even let you watch a class first, so you a can feel really comfortable with the "waters" before you jump in for a swim.

Don't put all your eggs in one yogic basket

Have you ever wondered how many snowflakes it takes to form three feet of fresh snow? Well, I don't know the specific answer, and that isn't the point anyway! The idea you need to grasp is that all those unique, individual snowflakes work together to create a perfect blanket of snow. The same is true of Power Yoga instructors. Every instructor is unique and each offers a different type of lesson that can benefit you in your Power Yoga practice.

After you find a good Power Yoga instructor, don't get the idea that you can't follow the practice of anyone else. No really good instructor asks you to swear off all other instructors anyway. Just as the ancient yogis learned by studying nature and its many lessons, your best method for learning Power Yoga is to find knowledge wherever it's available.

Find an instructor that you like, and rely on that person as your main teacher. Then, from time to time, attend classes with other instructors. You can expand your understanding of Power Yoga and bring something totally fresh and new to your practice.

If anything about the class seems uncomfortable for you, talk with the instructor to get all your questions answered. Then, if you're still not completely comfortable with the instructor, move on. And remember that some studios offer short-term classes that last for just a month or so. You may want to try one of these get acquainted deals before you commit to a long-term package.

Part III
Mastering the Basics

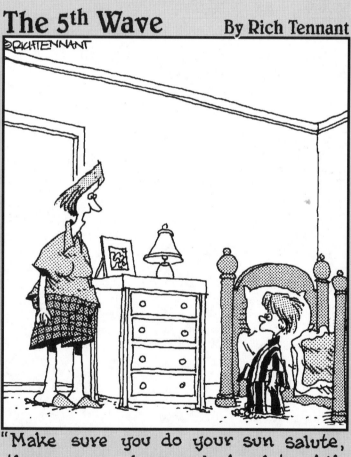

The 5th Wave   By Rich Tennant

"Make sure you do your sun salute, then your make-your-bed salute, while I go make your cereal salute."

In this part . . .

This part puts the *power* in Power Yoga. In these chapters, I show you how to sit, stand, and breathe in a Power Yoga way. I load you up on poses and the linking movements that make Power Yoga so powerful. I tell you how to warm up and how to cool down, and I give you three routines of varied lengths and difficulty. Get ready to turn on the power!

Chapter 7

Using Your Power Yoga Tools

*T*o really enjoy (and benefit from) your Power Yoga practice, you need to utilize some power tools of your own. I'm not talking about anything that requires an extension cord; I'm talking about making the most of your natural powers of breathing, muscle control, movement, focus, and body heat to really power up your Power Yoga routines.

I show you how to concentrate on each of these tools and develop it into the Power Yoga techniques of connecting links, focused gazing, muscle locks, and managed body heat. With the quick tour of your natural power tools' "user's manual" in this chapter, you'll be ready to launch into some basic Power Yoga routines.

Yoga Breathing Made Simple

You may be saying to yourself, "I know how to breathe. I don't need a book to tell me how to breathe." Well, believe it or not, to get the most from Power Yoga practice, you have to learn *Yoga breathing* — a technique of breath control called ujjayi. *Ujjayi*, which means "victorious breath," is quite different from regular breathing, but it isn't complicated. In fact, you can think of Yoga breathing as having three qualities:

> ✔ **A complete breath:** Taking a complete breath means to completely fill your lungs with air on an inhalation *(puraka)* and completely empty your lungs on an exhalation *(rechaka)*.

✔ **Slow, deep breathing:** In Yoga, your breathing is slow, deep, and rhythmic. Deep, controlled breathing corresponds with a calm and relaxed mind; it also enables you to take more oxygen into your lungs, leaving you feeling refreshed and invigorated.

✔ **Sound breathing:** Yoga breathing involves inhaling and exhaling air through your nose. As you breathe in through your nose, tighten the muscles in your throat slightly so that the incoming air makes a soft, hissing sound as if you're whispering the sound "Haaaaaaa". This tranquil, meditative sound, in combination with your slow, deep, measured breathing, contributes to the calming of your body and mind, enabling you to center your thoughts on your practice and ignore all other distractions.

Start Yoga breathing as you begin your practice and continue with the slow, fluid, rhythmic breathing until your practice is over. Learning breath control and the technique of ujjayi breathing offers several benefits:

✔ It oxygenates your blood and muscles.

✔ It brings fresh oxygen to your brain.

✔ It expands your lungs.

✔ It calms and relaxes your mind.

✔ It creates mental clarity.

✔ It creates abundant energy.

Practicing victorious Yoga breathing

Yoga breathing does more than just help you prepare for a role in the next *Star Wars* movie. It's an important part of Power Yoga's path to a calm, focused mind. To give this new breathing technique a whirl, try this fun ancient breathing exercise!

The curious sound of Yoga breathing

Question: What is the sound of ujjayi breathing?

(a) A vacuum cleaner

(b) Wind blowing through the mountains

(c) Darth Vader from *Star Wars*

Answer: All three! When you power breathe correctly, you may sound like any of these.

Feeding yourself the best energy

Prana, your vital life force, represents all the nutritional elements of earth, air, fire, water — all the elements that create life on this planet. Yoga practice helps you extract these elements from nature through your controlled breathing, to replenish the pranic energy within your own body and mind. Taking this concept one step further, many great Yoga masters have expressed the idea that air is a food. In theory, if you cleanse the body of toxins and live in a clean fresh environment, then air can serve as a supplemental nutritional source. The yogis believed that the best, most "nutritional" air is available near mountains, waterfalls, and oceans — areas in which the atmosphere is loaded with negatively charged ions. Practicing Yoga in areas in which you have a good supply of negatively charged ions is an incredibly powerful experience, as any Yoga practitioner knows. If you live near an area of natural splendor, step up to nature's lunch-counter and order a blue-plate special of high-quality, prana-enriching air! You'll be glad you did.

1. **Sit comfortably on the floor or in a chair.**

2. **Close your eyes and take a slow, deep breath through your nose.**

   Inhale fully, until your lungs feel completely expanded, and then slowly exhale through your nose. Your ujjayi breath is the human equivalent of a cat purring. Notice how your throat muscles have to tighten just a little bit to make the sound.

3. **Continue breathing slowly, deeply, and regularly, and with each inhalation and exhalation, slightly tighten your throat muscles as you feel and hear the air swirling past your throat.**

4. **With each exhalation, feel the air pass over the back of your throat and listen to the sound of your breath hissing past your throat and over the top of your mouth.**

   You know you've got it when you hear the light purring sound on both inhalation and exhalation and feel coolness at the back of your throat as you inhale.

Using Yoga breathing as a life force

You can use Yoga breathing in many areas of your daily life, not just during your Power Yoga workouts. Remember that Yoga teaches us that breath is your source of vital life force, so don't underestimate the powerful benefits of this seemingly simple tool. Your Yoga breathing technique can be a big help in these (and other) life situations:

- For relaxing in stressful situations
- For extending your physical endurance
- For bringing your mental clarity and focus to the finest pitch
- For quieting your mind, so you can enjoy peaceful rest
- For energizing your body and mind when you feel tired

I can offer you this guarantee of satisfaction as a reader of *Power Yoga For Dummies*. Use this Yoga breathing as a daily practice and as an emergency boost in stressful life situations. If you're not completely satisfied with the results, then go to your front door or window, exhale and send the air back where it came from. What more could you ask for in a no-risk free trial offer?

Power Yoga breathing versus traditional Yoga breathing

All forms of Yoga breathing are similar, but there are subtle differences. If you're a practitioner of traditional soft-form Yoga, it's important that you note a few critical differences between the Power Yoga breathing techniques you learn here and those of your current Yoga practice. With traditional Yoga breathing, you use the same complete Yoga breathing technique explained in this chapter. But in traditional Yoga breathing, you expand the lower abdominal muscles on inhalations and contract those muscles on exhalation.

In Power Yoga breathing, you keep your abdominal muscles firm and slightly contracted. When you inhale, you expand your chest and lift your rib cage. As you exhale, your chest sinks and your lungs contract. Your abdominal muscles remain engaged throughout the breathing cycle. The Power Yoga breathing technique is best for giving you strength and stability as you practice your poses, and this added stability can help you avoid injuries.

Controlling the Gateways of Internal Power (Energy Locks)

One of the important natural tools your body makes use of during Power Yoga practice is the *bandha,* or energy lock. You engage an energy lock by contracting certain muscles in your body; these contractions, or locks, direct through your body the flow of energy (the prana) that you create during Power Yoga exercises. Not only do energy locks help direct the flow of energy to high-demand areas during your Power Yoga practice, they also can give you energy boosts and added stability, and tone your stomach and cleanse your internal organs.

Understanding how energy locks work

To better understand the way energy locks work, visualize the workings of your circulatory system for a moment. Your heart pumps blood throughout your body, using your veins and arteries as the delivery system. When you practice Power Yoga, you create an enormous amount of life-force energy. This energy travels throughout your body through unseen channels called *nadis.* The energy locks act as valves to regulate the flow of life energy through the *nadis* in your body. In this respect, your bandhas work much like your heart, to control the flow of essential forces through your system.

Using muscle locks for a powerful practice

You should engage your energy locks each time you hold a Yoga asana or pose. You should release the bandha as you leave a pose, but often you re-engage the energy locks during your vinyasa, or linking movements.

Unlike the nadis (which you can't see), energy locks are made up of muscles groups in your body. To engage a bandha, you physically contract muscles in one of three areas of your body. Each of these three energy locks has a special name:

✔ **Mula bandha:** The *Mula bandha* is called the *root lock,* and it's located in the perineal muscles between your genitals and anus. To identify these muscles, imagine that you need to make an emergency trip to the bathroom and the nearest one is w-a-a-y down the hall. As you take that long walk, you engage your Mula bandha to fend off an unfortunate accident. Isn't that a great energy lock to have available?

✔ **Uddiyana bandha:** The name *uddiyana* means "flying up." This bandha is located about three-fingers width below your navel. In this bandha, you lift your stomach, drawing up your diaphragm. This bandha helps you look better in your bathing suit when you're at the beach, by flattening your stomach. In your Power Yoga practice, however, this bandha firms your abdominal muscles; you use it in conjunction with the Mula bandha.

✔ **Jalandhara bandha:** The jalandhara bandha is called a *chin lock.* You engage this bandha by stretching the back of the neck as you lower your chin into the notch in your breastbone. You engage this bandha in a few poses and in some Yoga breathing exercises, but you don't use it nearly as often as you use the Mula bandha or the Uddiyana bandha.

Figure 7-1 shows the location of these three bandhas.

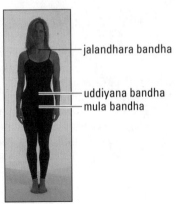

Figure 7-1: Engaging various muscle locks, or *bandhas,* helps turn up the power in your practice.

jalandhara bandha

uddiyana bandha
mula bandha

Making the Most of Vinyasas

Vinyasas, or connecting movements, link the power of your Power Yoga poses like electrical lines that carry power between generating stations. As you use a vinyasa to move from one pose to the next, you build upon the body heat and life-force energy that your exercises generate, and you maintain the power of your routine's momentum. The powerful conditioning and aerobic boost of the vinyasa connecting movements are what put the power in Power Yoga.

Moving with your breathing

Your breathing brings strength, vitality, and life to your vinyasa. As you move through your Power Yoga routines, always remember to move *with* your breathing. You can use your breathing to set the speed at which you move from one pose to the next. Use these guidelines for coordinating your breathing and movement during Power Yoga practice:

- ✔ As a general rule, exhale as you move into a Yoga posture, and inhale as you move out.
- ✔ Inhale when you are going against gravity, and exhale when you are going with gravity.
- ✔ Expand your chest as you inhale, and contract your chest as you exhale.
- ✔ Inhale before you move into a strength vinyasa, and then relax into the movement.

Using connecting links

In Power Yoga, you use connecting poses, or *vinyasas,* to enter and exit each posture, or *asana.* These connecting movements help you maintain the energy flow of your routine. For example, if you are in a seated posture and you need to go into a standing pose, you can scramble to your feet, tug at your workout clothes, and slowly shake yourself into position. The calm, gently flowing movement of a vinyasa, however, can transport you from one posture to the other with no break in energy, keeping the natural rhythm you've developed in your routine. Well-formed vinyasas make up the dance of Power Yoga. Do them correctly, and you're in *Swan Lake;* ignore them, and your routine is Funky Chicken all the way.

Some vinyasas are very strenuous. Because one function of the vinyasas is to generate body heat, strenuous vinyasas are referred to as *hot. Cool vinyasas* are less strenuous movements that you use to connect poses in the warm-up and cool-down phases of your Power Yoga routine.

Floating like a butterfly

As you move from one pose to the next during your Power Yoga workout, try to enter and exit each posture with grace and elegance. When I first learned Yoga, I moved between the poses like a clumsy bull. As I refined my technique, I came to think of each posture as a delicate flower. As I moved between them, I tried to float like a butterfly, so as not to disturb the calm beauty of the pose after I landed.

In all forms of Yoga, you develop power by developing softness. The smoother, gentler, and more controlled your movements are, the more they strengthen your body. And don't forget that the way you move has a big impact on your state of mind. When your body's jumping and jerking, your mind is twitchy and unsettled. But when you float like a butterfly, your mind is calm, relaxed, and in control.

Don't get me wrong; I expect you to be a bit awkward and uncoordinated when you first start practicing vinyasas and Power Yoga asanas. In the beginning, you're likely to move into vinyasas in spurts of speed. But as you gain experience, your Power Yoga practice improves in many ways — careful controlled movement is just one of the improvements you'll notice over time.

Time teaches you to go with the flow of your practice. Your practice becomes smooth and fluid and, ultimately, takes on the quality of a slow, soft dance. As you combine this gentle yet powerful movement with your deep breathing and mental focus, you gain the maximum Power Yoga benefit.

Finding points of focus (drishti)

This list includes the classic nine drishti used in traditional Yoga; the name of each drishti is followed by the place or thing on which you should focus your eyes when assuming this gazing point:

- **Nasagrai:** Tip of nose
- **Ajna Chakra:** Between the eyebrows
- **Nabi Chakra:** Your navel

- **Hastagrai:** Your hand
- **Padhayoragrai:** Your toes
- **Parsva Drishti:** Far to the side (either right or left)
- **Angustha Ma Dyai:** Your thumbs
- **Urvhva or Antara Drishti:** Up to the sky

Keeping your eyes on the Power Yoga prize

When I talk about "looking good" during Power Yoga, I don't mean wearing the right clothes, having the right hairstyle, or sporting the right genetic background. Nope, I'm referring to the way you direct your gaze as you move into and hold each Power Yoga posture. The way you direct and hold your gaze during Power Yoga practice has an impact on your mental state, your posture, and your ability to remain focused and energized.

In Yoga, the gazing point for each posture is called a *drishti,* which means both "looking out" and "looking in." The purpose of the drishti isn't to get your vision fixed on a particular place or part of your body; it's actually an exercise in turning your gaze inward. When you gaze inward, you can check to make sure that you're breathing properly, that your posture alignment is accurate, and that your energy lock is engaged. Gazing inward is a form of sense withdrawal, so your gaze is a tool to help you in this important part of Power Yoga practice. When you're "doing the drishti," you're focused: A gang of bikers could invade your Power Yoga studio, smoke cheap cigars, and gun their motorcycle engines, and you could go right on practicing without taking any notice of this unseemly distraction.

In most Power Yoga postures, you gaze in the direction of the posture's stretch. If you want to get technical about it and impress people at parties, you can memorize the focus or drishti gazing points listed in the "Finding points of focus" sidebar. Personally, I prefer not to be a fanatical drishti-ite and simply look in the direction of my stretch.

Benefiting from Body Heat

Power Yoga practice generates body heat. This body heat comes from the inside out, sort of like the heat that forms in a microwave oven. Your body heat is an important natural tool in Power Yoga. Body heat makes your muscles, tendons, and joints more pliable, and it makes you sweat. That sweat performs two powerful functions: It cools your body, and it helps remove toxins from your system.

Body heat is a tool that you really need to use correctly — or it can hurt you. Follow these guidelines to get the most benefit from the body heat that you generate during your Power Yoga workouts:

- ✔ As you sweat, you lose fluids, so drink lots of water before and after your Power Yoga practice.

- ✔ Try to work out in a warm (but not hot) room.

- ✔ If possible, have fresh air entering the room, but try to avoid blasts of cold air. Your muscles are most flexible in a warm environment, but quick changes in temperature can be damaging for your muscles (and your entire body, for that matter).

Putting All Your Power Tools to Work

It's one thing to read about how to practice Yoga breathing, energy locks, and points of gaze. But the real trick is learning to put them all to use while you're practicing a Power Yoga pose — especially one that requires lots of balance. But you can do it! And to show that I have complete confidence in you, I wrap up this chapter with an asana that requires you to pay special attention to balance. The Extended Foot One Leg Stand Posture (*utthita hasta padangusthasana*) trains you to incorporate all your natural tools into your Power Yoga practice.

In Sanskrit, the word *utthita* means "extended," *hasta* means "hand," and *padangustha* loosely translates to "big toe." In this posture, you stand on one leg while extending your other leg forward, grabbing your big toe with your hand.

The Extended Foot One Leg Stand Posture stretches and strengthens muscles in your legs, expands your chest, and opens those tight hips. In addition, this posture is wonderful for teaching balance and coordination. Follow these steps to perform this posture:

1. **Stand with your spine straight and your shoulders back, and extend your arms down the sides of your torso; keep your vision forward.**

   This is Mountain Pose I.

2. **Close your eyes for a few slow, deep yoga breaths while you maintain good posture.**

   Ground yourself firmly onto the floor, and be conscious and aware of your breathing.

3. **Open your eyes, and place your left hand on your left hip.**

4. **Pick your right foot up off the floor and, balancing on your left foot, bend your right knee and place your right hand around the outside of your right knee.**

   You should now be balancing on your left foot, holding your right knee with your right hand.

5. **Pull your right knee 90 degrees toward your right side as you open your hip.**

6. **Keep your torso and chest facing forward, and pull your right leg to your right side, turning your head to your left side and looking over your left shoulder (see Figure 7-2).**

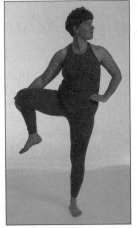

Figure 7-2:
This version of the Extended Foot One Leg Stand Posture is a great beginner's pose.

If you have trouble balancing, place your left hand on a wall for support.

7. **Put your power tools to work: Listen to the sound of your slow, deep breaths; engage your mula bandha by tightening your perineal muscles; engage your uddiyana bandha by firming and lifting your stomach; and direct your gaze (drishti) by looking over your left shoulder, parallel to the floor.**

8. **Hold this position for 5 to 10 slow deep breaths.**

9. **Release your energy locks, turn your head back to the center, and exhale as you bring your right leg back to the center and lower your foot to the floor.**

10. **Repeat these steps, but this time balance on your right leg, lift your left leg off the floor, and direct your drishti to the right.**

If you're an advanced student, you can do a full version of the Extended Foot One Leg Stand Posture by following the same series of steps, but instead of holding onto your knee, grab your right big toe with the first two fingers of your right hand and fully extend your leg out to the front and off to the side, as illustrated in Figure 7-3 (on the left side).

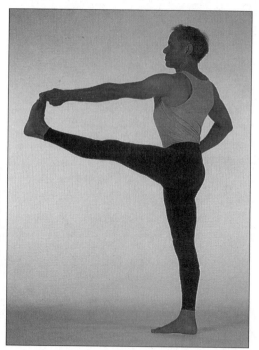

Figure 7-3:
Advanced students can try this version of the Extended Foot One Leg Stand Posture.

Chapter 8

Unfurling the Lotus and Other Seated Poses

. . . .

In This Chapter

▶ Practicing foundations for seated poses

▶ Using your best Power Yoga moves

▶ Moving beyond seated posture basics

▶ Helping your Full Lotus bloom

. . . .

In this chapter, I demonstrate the fundamental skills that you need for seated postures. I show you how to position your body, coordinate your breathing, and place your hands to get the greatest benefit from these important foundation poses. After reviewing the fundamentals, I give you some "beginner" postures, and then move through intermediate postures and the Half Lotus Posture to the Full Lotus and beyond.

When most people think of Yoga, they envision someone seated in the Lotus Posture. The Lotus Posture *(Padmasana)* is one of the most fundamental Yoga poses, and it gives you a good base for practicing breathing exercises and meditation. In fact, it's a good idea to allow time at the beginning and end of every Power Yoga session to sit quietly and breathe — in Lotus or any of the other seated postures that I present in this chapter.

When you use these postures correctly, you'll feel like a full-fledged yogi or yogini. So get ready to burst into flower — right where you're seated!

Getting Comfortable with Seated Postures

Like breathing, sitting down in Power Yoga isn't the same ol' thing that you know. You don't want to just dash into the seated poses like the winner in a round of musical chairs. To get the most from your entire Power Yoga routine, you need to understand the three must-know techniques for using seated postures:

- ✔ **Assuming the correct posture:** Making sure that your body is in the right position when you assume the seated posture is essential for benefiting from the exercise. Your posture affects your mental and physical readiness, your breathing, and your ability to focus. Don't worry, though; the instructions in this chapter are clear and simple, and they'll leave you sitting pretty.

- ✔ **Using Yoga breathing techniques:** Yoga breathing techniques are a central part of Power Yoga exercise. Using Yoga breathing helps you clear your mind, oxygenate your blood, maintain your focus, and get the most from your exercises. You really can't use the seated postures correctly unless you breath correctly. I remind you to use Yoga breathing in the instructions for each of the seated postures in this chapter, so if you need a refresher on the subject, check out the info in Chapter 7 or on the Cheat Sheet.

- ✔ **Placing your hands correctly:** In the ancient tradition of Yoga practice, the placement of your hands during seated postures symbolizes your efforts to unite your individual energy with the energy of the universe. I show you how to place your hands and fingers in jnana mudra, a symbolic gesture used in traditional meditation and practiced in the Lotus and many other seated postures.

Understanding these concepts makes practicing the seated postures easier, more comfortable, and more beneficial for your whole routine. Take a few moments to check out the following sections on these fundamentals, and your practice will be greatly rewarded.

Sitting simply: Basic seated postures

Remember when you were a kid and your mother was constantly harping on you to "straighten up" and "watch your posture"? Although you don't need to walk around balancing books on your head, you do have to watch the way you hold and position your body in Power Yoga. Your posture has a huge impact on the effectiveness of your Power Yoga practice. If you aren't in the correct posture, your breathing, mental clarity, and focus suffer. And the correct posture is critical for maintaining a stable base for your body — to help prevent injuries and fatigue.

By practicing a few simple, basic postures, you can become familiar with the "feel" of seated postures. And these simple postures are a good vehicle to incorporate the correct breathing techniques and hand gestures into your seated poses.

The Seated Angle Pose

This pose is a kind of launching pad for other postures and linking movements. Take the time to really concentrate on this pose — it's one of the basic seated postures that you'll use often in Power Yoga practice.

In this pose, your seated body forms a 90-degree angle (see Figure 8-1). The Seated Angle strengthens back muscles, promotes good posture, and creates a great foundation for transitions to other postures. You can use this posture for breath-control *(pranayama)* and meditation practice. Many people who have trouble with their knees find the Seated Angle to be a good alternative to the cross-legged seated poses.

This posture is most effective if you practice the Mula bandha and Uddiyana bandha muscle locks described in Chapter 7.

Figure 8-1:
The Seated Angle Pose is a great base for connecting to other Power Yoga exercises and sequences.

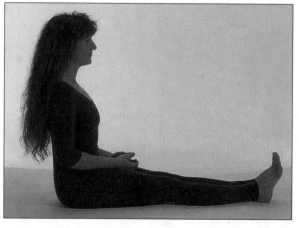

Follow these steps to use the Seated Angle Pose:

1. **Sit on the floor with both legs extended straight in front of you, your spine straight, and your shoulders back.**

2. **Keep your feet pointing upward and slightly flexed, as you fold your hands in your lap.**

   If your lower back is rounded, try placing a small pillow under your knees; this prop can help nudge your body into the proper posture.

3. **Hold this position for 5–10 slow deep breaths. Engage your muscle locks (see the Cheat Sheet).**

Easy Posture (Sukhasana)

Sukhasana means "pleasure or comfort," and in this posture, you can easily relax and be comfortable. If you're just getting into Yoga, the Easy Posture is a good preparation for learning the more complicated seated postures.

The Easy Posture, shown in Figure 8-2, promotes flexibility in your knees, ankles, and thighs, and contributes to giving you the excellent posture that your mother always dreamed you'd have!

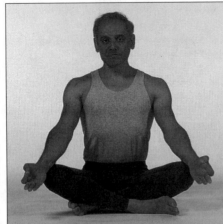

Figure 8-2:
The Easy Posture is traditionally used for breathing and meditation exercises.

Use these steps to practice the Easy Posture:

1. **Start from the Seated Angle Pose, sitting on the floor with your legs extended in front of you, your spine straight, and your shoulders back.**

2. **Bend your right knee, grasping your right ankle with your hands and pulling your foot toward your groin.**

   This forces your knee out to the side.

3. **Grasp your left ankle, and pull your left foot toward your groin, placing your left foot under your right knee.**

   You're now sitting cross-legged on the floor with your spine straight and your shoulders back. If you find this uncomfortable, place a small pillow under each knee.

   As an alternative for beginners, you can sit on a small pillow or on the edge of a chair. (Sitting on the edge of the chair keeps your back straight.) Make sure that the chair is solid enough to be stable when you sit on the front edge.

4. **Extend your arms, and rest your wrists and hands on your knees, with palms facing upward, and form Jnana Mudra (see Figure 8-4).**

5. **Hold this position for 5–10 slow, deep Power Yoga breaths (see the Cheat Sheet), remembering to close your eyes, calm your mind, and relax.**

Persuading Posture Trainer

To help you incorporate the basics of a good seated posture, I present to you the Personal Posture Trainer (see Figure 8-3). The name is fitting because it helps you to overcome bad posture habits, and it relieves stress and tension in your shoulders and arms. Try this exercise after a hard day's work. It's a good way to relax and get your body and head straight.

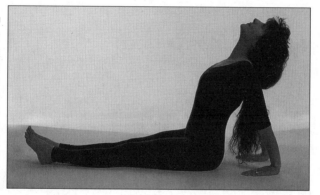

Figure 8-3: The Persuading Posture Trainer lets you experience the feeling of sitting correctly.

Use these steps to practice the Persuading Posture Trainer:

1. **Sit on the floor in either the Easy Posture or Seated Angle Pose. (Refer to Figure 8-1 or Figure 8-2.)**

2. **Rest your hands in your lap, keeping your spine straight and your shoulders back; relax and take a few slow, deep breaths.**

3. **Extend your arms behind your torso, fingers facing forward, bend your elbows, and place your palms on the floor.**

4. **Slide your hands backward — about 2 feet behind you so that your arms are fully extended but your elbows aren't locked. Expand your chest and allow your torso to lean backward.**

5. **Keep your vision forward and hold this position for 2 to 5 deep breaths; relax, placing you hands back into your lap, and repeat Steps 2 through 5.**

Practicing Yoga breathing techniques in Seated Postures

Your breathing is a simple, yet complex function that you practice subconsciously throughout your life. Yoga breathing is very simple. Still, you do have to get used to the technique of breathing in and out through your nose; filling and emptying your lungs completely as you inhale and exhale. You also may need a bit of practice to produce the curious sound of Yoga breathing — the purring noise that results from pushing the air over the back of your throat.

You get the most from every seated posture when you remember to incorporate your Yoga breathing technique. Check out the Cheat Sheet if you need more information on the breathing technique itself.

Handling your hands with the Jnana Mudra

Many seated poses require specific placement of your hands and fingers, called *Jnana Mudra*. In Sanskrit, *jnana* means "knowledge" or "wisdom," and a *mudra* is a "seal" or "lock." Traditionally, many yogis and yoginis use Jnana Mudra as they meditate and as part of many seated postures.

Everything about this gesture has symbolic meaning. In Jnana Mudra, your index finger represents your soul, and your thumb represents the universe. As you unite the tip of your thumb with the tip of your index finger, you symbolically unite the energy of your soul with that of the universe, thereby tapping into the wisdom of the entire universe.

Use these steps to achieve the Jnana Mudra:

1. **Sit on the floor in the Easy Posture.**

   You may also use any other seated posture described in this chapter.

2. **Place your hands on your knees with your palms facing upward.**

3. **Open your hands, and bend your index finger in to touch the tip of your thumb.**

   Your remaining fingers should be straight, but not stiff or tense. See Figure 8-4.

4. **Hold this hand placement as you remain in the seated posture and practice Yoga breathing for 5–10 breaths.**

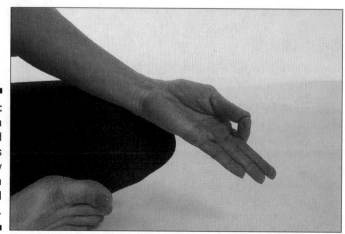

Figure 8-4:
The Jnana
Mudra hand
gesture is
part of many
Power Yoga
seated
postures.

Building a Seated Posture Repertoire

The seated poses in this chapter are a foundation for your entire Power Yoga practice. Because seated postures are so central to Power Yoga, you need to practice them carefully. In this section, I give you an opportunity to gradually sprout your lotus petals. Here, you discover some of the preliminary seated postures and practice some gentle stretching exercises that can help prepare you for the somewhat more demanding Full Lotus Posture, which I describe later in the chapter.

Each person has a unique body, so you may find that the Easy Posture is very comfortable for you, while the Kneeling Posture is more comfortable for me. The following seated postures offer something for everyone: Some of them are cross-legged postures, some are kneeling postures, and others are extended-leg seated postures. The best training technique is to find a seated posture that you're comfortable with, and use it as your base. Then, a few times a week, alternate trying some of the other seated postures that you need to practice.

When you're learning a new physical exercise, you can expect to experience some discomfort. That discomfort is a natural result of challenging your body to get into shape. But persistent pain (especially joint pain) is your body's way of telling you to back off. You have to decide when to push and when to stop pushing, but always listen to your body. With any of these seated postures, you want to avoid injuries to your knees. Take your time, try the alternative postures, and if it feels right for you, great. But don't push yourself beyond reasonable limits.

Drive the Lotus, don't let it drive you

It's a good idea to master as many seated postures as you can and to use a number of them in your Power Yoga routine. Many consider the Full Lotus to be the ultimate seated posture and a must for any yogi or yogini. But don't get caught up in Lotus mania. You don't *have* to practice the Full Lotus Posture at all; any of the seated postures in this chapter are fine alternatives. Your body may not be as adaptable to the Full Lotus Position as you would like, and you can damage your knees by trying to force your body into this posture. The fact is, if you are a real yogi or yogini, then you know how to listen to your body, and you do whatever it takes to preserve your precious machine. So grab a seated posture — any one will do!

Remember that your knee joint is one of the more vulnerable joints in your body. Although there are now reasonable replacements, nothing works quite as well as your original equipment. The real movement of your knee to the floor needs to come from your hip. So if you try to get your knees to the floor before your hips open, you threaten the stability of your knees — and depending on what you try, you may be unkind to your ankles also. Not a good idea. So practice Power Yoga preparation poses with patience and persistence. Rely on your body, not your mind, to tell you when you're ready for the full Lotus.

Riding a Thunderbolt (Vajrasana)

The Sanskrit word *vajra* means "thunderbolt," but this posture is sometimes called Hero or Champion. The Thunderbolt stimulates the nerves in your feet and lower legs, and stretches the muscles in your feet and ankles. In fact, many Yoga masters use this pose to correct flat feet and strengthen arches. This pose is a good alternative for the cross-legged poses, and it's a common base posture for breathing and meditation.

Use these steps to practice the Thunderbolt Pose:

1. **Gently kneel on the floor, keeping your spine straight and shoulders back.**

   You may want to use your yoga mat. Padding is often important in this pose, especially for those who have had knee problems.

2. **Sit back on your heels, with your toes pointed backward; feel your neck lengthen, and then fold your hands in your lap.**

3. **Gaze straight head, parallel to the floor.**

4. **Hold this position for 5–10 complete breaths.**

   See Figure 8-5 for an illustration of this pose.

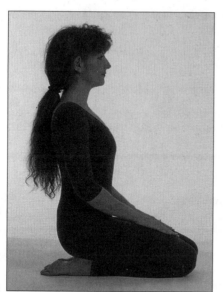

Figure 8-5:
The
Thunderbolt
Pose.

If you have knee problems, try placing a rolled towel or small pillow between your calves and thighs, locating the prop where it feels most comfortable. The prop eases the pressure and can make the Thunderbolt Pose more comfortable.

Finding the Perfect Posture (Siddhasana)

In Sanskrit, *siddha* means "perfect." A siddha is also a great prophet or sage, one who is very pure and spiritual, and whose perfection has resulted in magical powers. This pose was practiced more than 5,000 years ago by ancient Yoga sages, many of whom considered it to be the perfect posture for breath control practice *(pranayama)* and meditation exercises. As you practice the Perfect Posture, you're connecting with the wisdom of those ancient Yoga masters. Be sure to bring your pure and spiritual side along as you enjoy this pose and see what magic this posture can bring.

The Perfect Posture, shown in Figure 8-6, helps open your chest and limber up your ankles, knees, and thighs. It is more advanced than the Easy Posture and promotes more flexibility in your leg muscles.

Use these steps to practice the Perfect Posture:

1. **Sit cross-legged on the floor, bending your knees and pulling both heels in snug to the base of your torso.**

2. **Gently lower both knees to the floor.**

   If you feel any discomfort in your lower back, lift your hips a bit by sitting on a small pillow or folded blanket. Try not to round your lower back.

3. **Extend your arms over your thighs, and rest your hands on your knees in the Jnana Mudra Position.**

   Remember to keep your spine straight, and embrace good posture.

4. **Hold this position for five slow, deep breaths. Try to practice engaging the Mula bandha and Uddiyana bandha muscle locks.**

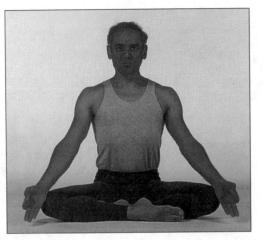

Figure 8-6:
The Perfect Posture is a powerful exercise for promoting flexible ankles, knees, and thighs.

Floating into the Butterfly Pose (Baddha Konasana)

I call this pose the Butterfly, because the movement of your thighs and knees resembles a butterfly softly landing on a flower. The quite unlovely name — as translated from the Sanskrit — is "caught or bound" *(baddha)* "angle" *(kona)* "pose" *(asana)*. Don't you like my name for it better?

The Butterfly Pose is wonderful for opening the hips, stretching out the muscles of the thighs, and creating flexibility in the ankles. The posture also helps increase the blood supply to your abdomen and pelvis.

Use these steps to practice the Butterfly Pose:

1. **Sit on the floor in the Seated Angle Pose, with your legs stretched out in front of you.**

2. **Bend your knees, bringing your feet in toward the base of your torso, with knees out to your sides and the soles of your feet facing each other.**

3. **Try to bring the soles of your feet together, as you lock your intertwined fingers around both feet.**

4. **Maintain good posture as you let gravity take your thighs toward the floor.**

5. **Lean forward, trying to bring your abdomen out over your feet.**

   Figure 8-7 shows you what this should look like.

6. **Hold this position for 5–10 complete breaths.**

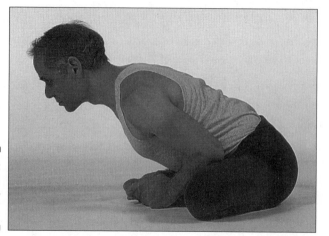

Figure 8-7: The Butterfly Pose.

Moving up to the Half Lotus Posture (Ardha Padmasana)

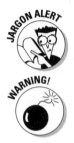

In Sanskrit, *ardha* means "half" and *padma* means "lotus." In this posture, you're halfway to the Full Lotus Posture. This pose, illustrated in Figure 8-8, helps invigorate the nerves in your legs and thighs; it also helps loosen up your hip and knee joints, and increases flexibility in your ankles.

With Full Lotus and Half Lotus, you must practice in moderation, or you risk damage to the knees. (See the section, "Blooming into Full Lotus," for precautions you should take.)

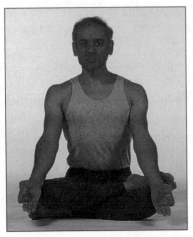

Figure 8-8:
The Half Lotus Posture gets you on your way to the Full Lotus and can be a fine seated asana on its own.

Use these steps to practice the Half Lotus Posture:

1. **Sit on the floor in the Easy Posture (refer to Figure 8-2), with your legs crossed and your breathing calm.**

   Your body and mind should be relaxed.

2. **Take your right foot in your hands, and gently place your right ankle on top of your left thigh.**

   Try to align your right heel with your hip joint while keeping your ankle straight.

3. **Extend your arms over your knees, and place your hands in Jnana Mudra Position.**

4. **Close your eyes, and hold this position for 5–10 slow deep breaths.**

5. **Try to engage your Mula bandha and Uddiyana bandha.**

6. **Relax for a moment, and then change the position of your legs by returning your right leg to its original Easy Posture, and gently placing your left ankle on top of your right thigh.**

7. **Close your eyes, and hold this position for 5–10 deep breaths.**

8. **Open your eyes, gently take your left ankle off your right thigh, return to your Easy Posture, and relax.**

Watering Your Lotus

Doing this exercise, you look like a parent gently rocking a baby. By practicing the Watering Your Lotus Posture, you open your hips and create more flexibility in your lower legs. This is a good preparation for the Lotus Posture.

Use these steps to practice the Watering Your Lotus Posture:

1. **Sitting on the floor in the seated pose of your choice, bend your left knee and cradle your leg with your arms, pulling your leg into your chest, as if you were holding a baby. Try to bring your leg to a 90-degree angle. Sit up tall, keeping your spine long.**

2. **Hold this position, and start taking slow, deep breaths.**

3. **Rock your bent leg (your "baby") from right to left with a gentle, smooth motion, as you continue your slow, deep breathing.**

4. **On an exhalation, pull your left bent leg toward your chest — up as high toward your shoulders as possible — and hold for a few breaths (see Figure 8-9).**

5. **Lower your leg to the floor, and repeat Steps 1 through 4 with the left leg.**

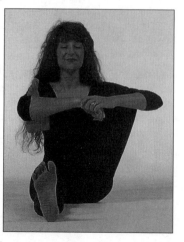

Figure 8-9:
The Watering Your Lotus Posture helps increase flexibility in your hips and lower legs.

If the cross-legged sitting postures hurt your knees or lower back, don't force your body to endure the pain. Remember that you're practicing Yoga to ease pain, not cause it! So if the seated poses hurt, try some props. For example, you can sit on a pillow or folded blanket, and place small pillows under your bent knees so that your legs are supported. And if the floor just won't work for you at all, you can practice many seated postures sitting on the edge of a chair. You can also try this pose on your back, with your uncradled foot on the floor close to your seat, knee toward the ceiling. This position protects your lower back and still gives you all the movement in your hip. Use these suggestions to help begin practicing the seated postures; in a few weeks or months, you may be able to drop the props!

Blooming into Full Lotus (And Beyond)

The Full Lotus Posture is a wonderful exercise for opening up the hips and creating flexibility in the ankles and knees. Practiced in moderation, the Lotus can invigorate the nerves of your legs and thighs. I have personally found that the strength and flexibility I've gained by practicing the Lotus Posture has helped me to avoid injuries when I'm partaking in other activities, such as hiking and skiing.

Proceeding with caution

The Full Lotus is a very advanced pose, so be extremely aware of your knees and take your time as you move into the Lotus Posture. This posture is too much of a stretch for you if you feel pain in your knees or lower back. Practice first with the alternative seated postures and exercises earlier in this chapter. As your flexibility improves, you can continue to try the Full Lotus Position until it feels comfortable and right for you. Until then, don't push your body into this posture.

Even when you feel comfortable assuming the Full Lotus Posture, let your Lotus bloom slowly — knees are a precious commodity, so give them some respect. Your ligaments and joints accept gradual changes. If you use this posture too much, or too soon, you could badly injure your knees and slow the progress of your entire Power Yoga practice.

Low-down on the Lotus Posture

The Lotus Posture is named for the lotus flower — a type of water lily that has multiple petals and floats on ponds and slow streams. When you see a real lotus flower, up close and personal, you understand how this posture inherited its name. The lotus flower possesses a calm, quiet beauty that yoga practitioners can contemplate — and mirror — in this seated posture.

Because the lotus has its roots in the muck of the lake or pond bottom and its blooms face toward heaven, because it moves with the water yet doesn't lose its rooting, it is the perfect symbol of the Yoga practice that is both grounded and spiritually oriented.

Part of the power and effectiveness of the Lotus Position comes from the triangle shape your body assumes. Many Eastern cultures believe that a triangular shape, such as those of the pyramids of Egypt, harnesses life energy. Triangles also symbolize knowledge, will, and action, three key aspects of your Power Yoga practice. By turning your body into a mini-pyramid, you can tap into this mystical energy and stay very grounded at the same time.

For many years, I thought that in order to be a real yogi, I had to do the Lotus Posture. Yet for almost a year, I had problems with my knees. Then I learned to move slowly and gradually coax my knees into accepting this posture. Benefit from my lesson, and take the Lotus in small steps; then you'll enjoy healthy knees and a long, active Power Yoga practice.

Practicing the Full Lotus (Padmasana)

The word *padma* means "lotus." In this posture, you float like a water lily as you create the beauty of a lotus flower with your body and in your mind. The Lotus Posture is a classic pose for meditation and pranayama, controlled Yoga breathing. Another name for this posture is the Buddha Pose; many yogis and yoginis, past and present, envision the Buddha meditating in this pose.

If you want a less challenging alternative to the Full Lotus Pose, try using the Easy Posture.

Use these steps to practice the Full Lotus Posture:

1. **Sit on the floor in the Easy Posture.**

   Your back is straight, your mind is calm, and you are completely focused and relaxed.

2. **Take your right foot in your hands, and slowly place it on your left thigh as close to the crease of your hip as you can.**

   Try to align your left heel with your hip joint while keeping your left ankle straight.

3. **Take your left foot in your hands, and slowly place it on your right thigh as close to the crease of your hip as you can.**

   Try to align your right heel with your hip joint while keeping your right ankle straight.

4. **Be aware of correct posture as you open your chest, lengthen your spine, and gently pull your shoulders back; feel yourself relax as you sit proud, with your chin held high.**

   Remember to press in at your lower back to maintain its natural inward curve.

5. **Extend your arms over your thighs, and rest your hands and wrists on your knees, with palms facing upward.**

6. **Place your hands in the Jnana Mudra Position.**

   You now are in the Full Lotus Position, as illustrated in Figure 8-10.

7. **Close your eyes and hold this pose for 5–10 slow deep breaths.**

    Calm your mind and relax, as you feel yourself gently floating.

8. **As you breathe, try to engage the Mula bandha and Uddiyana bandha muscle locks.**

    You may even try jalandara bandha, in this pose. (For a review of the bandhas see Chapter 7 or the Cheat Sheet.)

9. **Open your eyes; take your left ankle in your hands and slowly lower your left foot to the floor, and then take your right ankle in your hands and lower your right foot to the floor.**

10. **Relax for a few breaths in the Easy Posture.**

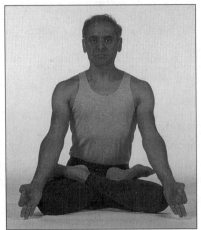

Figure 8-10:
The Full
Lotus.

The next time you practice this posture, place your left foot on your right thigh first. Alternating the order of your foot placement each time you assume the Lotus Position, gives your muscles a balanced stretch over the course of your Power Yoga practice.

Sampling the beginning Bound Lotus (with props)

After you've tackled the Full Lotus Position and feel perfectly comfortable with it, you may want to try a posture that takes you just a bit further down the Power Yoga road. The Bound Lotus Posture (Baddha Padmasana) is just the ticket; it gives you all the benefits of the Full Lotus, along with some wonderful expansion and stretches for the muscles of your chest. *Padma* means "lotus" and *baddha* means, "caught or bound." In this posture, you take hold of your feet by wrapping your arms and hands around behind your lower back and trying to grasp your toes; this wrapping action binds the Lotus and closes the energy loop within the body.

The Bound Lotus is a very difficult pose to accomplish; often, body type determines whether you can be successful with this posture. The full variation (without props) is tremendously advanced, which is why I offer it as the last exercise in this chapter. But if you feel like giving this posture a whirl, why not start out with this modified version, using props?

In this version of the Bound Lotus, you use straps (or even long towels) as props to extend your reach (see Figure 8-11). This beginner's version of the Bound Lotus is an excellent alternative for first-timers to this advanced posture.

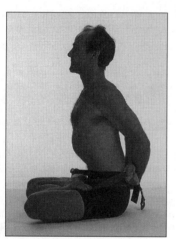

Figure 8-11:
The Bound
Lotus (with
props).

Use these steps to practice the Bound Lotus Posture (with the help of props):

1. **Sit on the floor in the Easy Posture.**

   Your back is straight, your mind is calm, and you are completely focused and relaxed.

2. **Place your left foot up on your right thigh.**

3. **Wrap a Yoga strap around your left ankle, and place the other end of the strap behind your lower back.**

   A Yoga strap works best, but you can use a towel, a tie, or a cloth belt.

4. **Grasp the strap with your left hand behind your lower back.**

5. **Place your right foot on your left thigh, and wrap a strap around your right ankle.**

6. **Place the other end of this Yoga strap behind your lower back, and grasp it with your right hand behind your lower back.**

   Refer to Figure 8-11 for an illustration of using these straps.

7. **Hold this position for 5 slow, deep breaths with your eyes closed.**

   Try to practice engaging Mula bandha and Uddiyana bandha.

8. **Open your eyes, and release your hands from the straps.**

9. **Take your right ankle in your hands, and gently lower your right foot to the floor; then take your left ankle in your hands, and lower your left foot to the floor.**

10. **Take the straps off your ankles, and relax into the Easy Posture.**

As you practice the Bound Lotus (with or without props) more frequently in your Power Yoga routines, try to alternate which foot you first move onto your thigh to balance the effect of this posture on your body.

Going all the way in the Bound Lotus (Baddha Padmasana)

When you're ready for the big kahuna, try this full version of the Bound Lotus. This pose is wonderful for teaching your body to naturally assume good posture. Because you wrap your arms behind your back in the Bound Lotus, you expand your chest and lift your shoulders. This helps to pull your body into proper alignment, with your back straight, your shoulders back, and your chest held full and high. The Bound Lotus leaves you feeling refreshed and energetic, and it relieves tension in your torso.

Remember that this is a *very advanced* posture; proceed slowly and pay attention to your own limits.

Use these steps to practice the Bound Lotus Posture (without props):

1. **From the Full Lotus Posture, reach behind your back with your left hand and grasp the toes of your left foot.**

   If necessary, lean forward until you can take hold of your toes.

2. **Reach behind your back with your right hand to grasp toes of your right foot.**

3. **Sit up gradually, maintaining correct posture.**

   See Figure 8-12 for an illustration of this posture.

It's not possible to maintain correct posture while you transition into this posture; after you grasp your feet, however, your body will correct itself into the proper alignment.

4. **Close your eyes, relax into this posture, and hold for 5–15 complete slow, deep breaths.**

   Try to practice engaging Mula bandha and Uddiyana bandha.

5. **Open your eyes, and release the grip of your hands on your toes.**

6. **Grasp your right ankle, and slowly lower your right foot to the floor; then grasp your left ankle, and slowly lower your left foot to the floor.**

7. **Relax into the Easy Posture.**

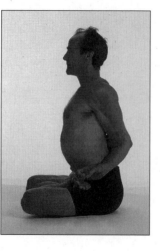

Figure 8-12:
The Bound
Lotus
without
props.

Chapter 9

Preparing with Powerful Warm-Ups

In This Chapter

▶ Finding ground zero with floor-based warm-ups

▶ Feeding the tiger in your tank

▶ Standing up to your warm-ups

I'm sure that you never drive your car without first warming up the engine. Everyone knows that a cold engine is a poor performer, subject to backfiring and stalling out. Well, the wonderful machine that you call your body doesn't run smoothly without a warm-up, either. If you want your body to function at full capacity, with limber joints, flexible muscles, and energy to spare, you need to take time to warm 'er up before any strenuous activity — and that definitely includes your Power Yoga workouts. Even the most advanced Power Yoga practitioners take time to warm up before launching into a fast-paced Power Yoga session.

In this chapter, I share some of my favorite warm-up routines. I divided the warm-ups into two sections: warm-ups practiced on the floor (lying down, sitting, or kneeling) and standing warm-ups.

Getting Down with Warm-Ups on the Floor

These gentle warm-ups are designed to gradually speed up the circulation of your whole body, through balanced stretches and counter-stretches. (A *counter-stretch* stretches the opposite side of the body or muscle, as the case may be. For example, the counter-stretch for a forward bend is a backward bend.) As an added bonus, these warm-ups help you develop coordination and balance as they take you through twists, turns, and stretches.

Twisting with the Spine Toner

The Spine Toner is relaxing, easy to practice, and a great way to flex your spine. Your everyday routines — work, play, even sitting — can deliver lots of abuse to your spine. This simple warm-up helps your spine recuperate from its long, hard days.

The Spine Toner invigorates your entire spine with gentle twisting movements that stretch the muscles in your back and hips. To get the most from this warm-up, be sure to combine it with the Power Yoga breathing techniques described in Chapter 7 and repeated on the Cheat Sheet.

Follow these steps to tone your spine:

1. **Lie down on the floor on your back, with your legs straight and your feet about 12 inches apart (a position known as the Corpse Posture — see the Cheat Sheet), and extend your arms straight out from your shoulders at a 90-degree angle from your torso.**

2. **On an inhalation, bend your right knee and lift your right leg toward the ceiling, exhale, and then lower your right leg over your left leg toward the floor, on the left side of your body. Then extend your leg fully to the side.**

   Keep your legs straight, but not rigid. If you find this posture uncomfortable, keep your right knee bent.

3. **Your right hip will automatically rise off the floor, and your whole torso will twist, but try to keep your shoulders flat on the floor as you turn your head and gaze to the right.**

   Figure 9-1 illustrates what this pose looks like.

4. **Hold this position for 5–15 slow deep breaths, and then slowly lift your right leg and return it to its original position (see Step 1).**

5. **Repeat Steps 1 through 4, this time using your left leg and gazing toward the left in Step 3.**

6. **Relax in the Corpse Posture for 5–10 slow, deep breaths.**

Hey, astronaut, you're walking upside-down

Even for a complete novice this exercise is easy and fun. In this pose, you look like someone who's walking upside down — and you don't require a zero-gravity chamber! This exercise delivers many of the same benefits to your body that you get from walking right side up. The Upside-Down Walker is an excellent warm-up exercise; it speeds up your circulation, stretches your arms and legs, and helps send a fresh supply of blood to the brain.

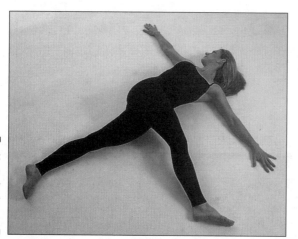

Figure 9-1:
The Spine
Toner gently
twists your
spine.

Follow these steps to walk upside down:

1. **Lie flat on your back, with your arms and legs straight, but not rigid.**

2. **Stretch your arms and legs upward, pointing toward the ceiling, like a bug stuck on its back.**

3. **Now swing you're arms and legs as though you are walking in the air (see Figure 9-2).**

   If you have stiff leg muscles and tight hips, bend your knees more to protect your lower back from overstrain.

   Swing your left arm forward (toward your face), when your right leg is forward; then swing your right arm forward when your left leg is forward.

4. **Take 15–30 strides.**

5. **Return your arms and legs to the floor, and relax in your original position.**

Make sure to move your limbs in opposite directions — move your right arm and left leg at the same time and your left arm and right leg together.

Hugging those knees

Your knees are responsible for lots of work and some of your most important moves; here's your chance to thank them for all their effort! In this exercise, you pay tribute to your knees by giving them a big hug.

This exercise relieves tension in your lower back, expands your chest, and tones up your stomach muscles. And as an added bonus, these knee hugs can also help relieve your system of excessive gas — something for which everyone can be grateful.

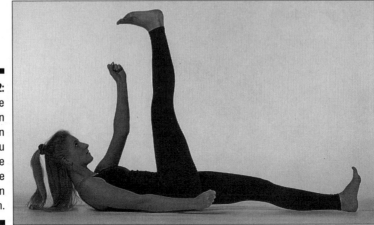

Figure 9-2:
The Upside
Down
Walker can
make you
feel like
you're
walking on
the moon.

Hug your knees close to you with these steps:

1. **Lie down on your back, with arms by your sides, palms facing up and legs extended.**

   Leave your feet about one foot apart.

2. **Calm your mind, and relax for a few slow, deep breaths.**

   This is called the Corpse Position.

3. **On an inhalation, stretch your whole body in both directions, lifting your arms above your head and stretching your legs out from your feet. Keep your head on the floor and gaze upward.**

4. **Exhale, and lower your arms toward your waist, while bending your right knee into your torso, wrapping your arms around your shin, and hugging your right knee.**

   If you have a weak lower back, bend your extended left leg, knee raised upward and place your left foot on the floor about two feet from your seat.

5. **On an exhalation, lift your head off the floor and try to touch your nose to your knee.**

6. **Inhale, and release your knee, again stretching your whole body in both directions.**

   Lift your arms over your head, and stretch your legs toward your feet.

7. **Repeat this action 3–5 times.**

8. **Relax as you lower your arms to your sides and melt softly into the floor, returning to the Corpse position (refer to Step 1).**

9. **Repeat the same exercise, following Steps 3 through 7, hugging your left knee this time.**

10. **Relax into the Corpse Position.**

Another way to ease the strain on your lower back is to bend your downward knee — point your knee toward the ceiling with your foot 12 to 18 inches from your seat. Keeping your knee bent reduces the intensity of the effort required and is gentler on your lower back.

Releasing shoulder and neck tension

Who can resist a nice shoulder and neck massage? All day, you build tension and stress in your neck and shoulders, and by the end of the day you need a massage — and you need it in the worst way! The problem is that you also need a willing masseuse. Well, these two exercises let you give *yourself* a massage to roll the tension right out of those tight neck and shoulder muscles.

These exercises are also terrific warm-ups for your Power Yoga routines. Give them a try before your Power Yoga workout or anytime you need to roll the weight of the world off your shoulders.

Rolling the boulders off your shoulders

"Row, row, row your boat, gently down the stream," goes the song. Wouldn't that hurt with your shoulders feeling as tight as they do right now? You need strong, healthy shoulders to excel in Power Yoga, so this shoulder roll exercise can be an important preamble to your workout.

In this exercise, you lift and lower your shoulders while rotating them in forward and backward circles. These shoulder rolls help you release tension from your shoulders and upper back, and get your rotator cuff (where your arm connects into your torso) warmed up and ready for action.

Follow these steps to get your shoulders rolling:

1. **Sit on the floor, with your spine straight and shoulders back (see the Seated Angle Pose on the Cheat Sheet).**

   If sitting on the floor is uncomfortable for you, you also can sit on the edge of a sturdy chair.

2. **On an inhalation, rotate your shoulders backward as you lift them up toward your ears.**

3. **As you exhale, finish the backward rotation as you lower your shoulders to their original position.**

4. **Repeat this action, reversing the direction of your shoulder rotation.**

5. **Repeat each rotation three or four times, and then relax your shoulders.**

Getting rid of that pain in the neck

When the muscles in your neck get tight and stiff, they can interfere with all your upper body movements. This exercise knocks the kinks out of stiff necks to get you warmed up and ready for action.

This exercise helps you to release stress and tension from your neck, stimulating the nerves in your upper spine and the base of your skull. This simple but powerful exercise is also a great way to build strength and flexibility in all the muscles in your neck, leaving you less prone to future attacks of neck stiffness and pain. Best of all, this exercise is very relaxing.

Follow these steps to warm up your neck muscles:

1. **Sit on the floor (or on the edge of a sturdy chair) with your spine straight and your shoulders back; relax your arms and rest your hands in your lap.**

2. **On an exhalation, tilt your head forward and let your chin drop to your chest.**

   You feel the muscles in the back of your neck stretch.

3. **Inhale, and lift your head back to its upright position.**

4. **Exhale, and tilt your head back as far as you can without hurting anything.**

   You feel the muscles in the front of your neck and under your chin stretch.

5. **Again, inhale and return your head to its upright position.**

6. **Repeat Steps 1 through 5 four times, and then return to your original posture.**

7. **Exhale, and lower your head to your right shoulder; inhale and raise your head to its original position.**

8. **Repeat this action, but lower your head to the left side on an exhalation and back to center on an inhalation.**

9. **Relax for three complete breaths.**

   Use your Yoga breathing technique for maximum benefit.

10. **On an exhalation, turn your head to the right; keep your head level as you gaze over your right shoulder; inhale and turn your head to look straight ahead.**

11. **Repeat this action, turning your head and gazing to the left on an exhalation and back to center on an inhalation.**

12. **Finish by closing your eyes and relaxing for three complete breaths.**

Playing with the kitty (Cat Stretch)

The movements of this exercise resemble a cat stretching out the kinks after a good long sleep. The Cat Stretch is an excellent exercise for almost anyone and a great substitute for the Sun Salutation that I describe in Chapter 10.

The Cat Stretch tones up your back muscles and can make your entire spine feel stronger and more flexible. If you suffer from minor back pain brought on by stress, over-activity, or bad posture, this exercise can help relieve that pain and get you back in action.

Follow these steps to imitate your cat:

1. **Start from a kneeling position; sit back on your heels, with your toes pointed backward, your back straight, and your neck lengthened, with your head facing forward.**

2. **Lift your hips, and place your hands on the floor, so that you're resting on your hands and knees.**

3. **Keep your back straight, but not rigid, and relax as you take three slow, deep breaths.**

   Your body forms a table in this pose, as shown in Figure 9-3.

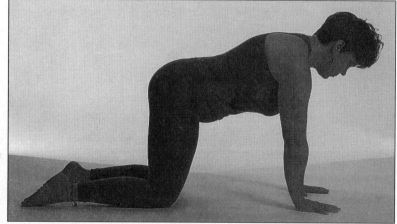

Figure 9-3:
The Table
Pose.

4. **On an exhalation, arch your back like a cat.**

5. **Relax your neck as you drop your head downward and gaze toward your knees, as illustrated in Figure 9-4.**

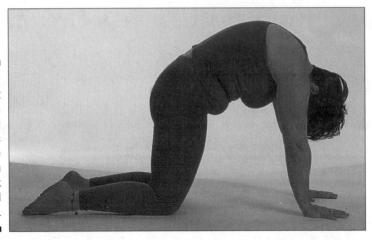

Figure 9-4:
The Cat
Stretch with
an arched
back helps
loosen the
muscles in
your back
and
shoulders.

6. On an inhalation, lower your back, expanding your chest, and let your back arch downward as you bend your arms to lower your chest and bring your chin to rest on the floor between your hands, as shown in Figure 9-5.

7. Exhale, and slowly draw your body up to return to the arched-back position you entered in Step 3.

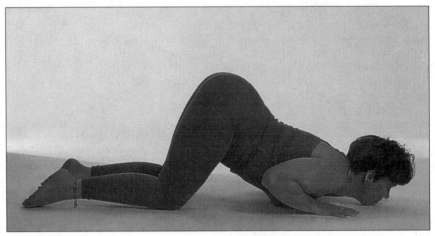

Figure 9-5:
The Cat
Stretch with
a swayed
back helps
relieve
tension in
your spine.

8. On an inhalation, sway your back downward again, but keep your arms straight and lift your head up as you extend your right leg back and up.

   If your back is arched properly and your leg and head are extended up, your body forms a smile in this phase of the Cat Stretch, as shown in Figure 9-6.

Don't swing or jerk into this posture: Try to keep your movements fluid and soft as you lift your head and extend your leg back and up.

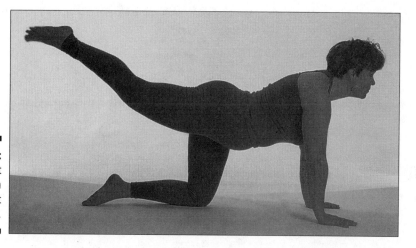

Figure 9-6:
The Cat Stretch with the right leg back.

9. **On an exhalation, reverse the stretch; arch your back again and drop your head, bending your right knee into your chest.**

   Try to touch your nose with your knee, as illustrated in Figure 9-7.

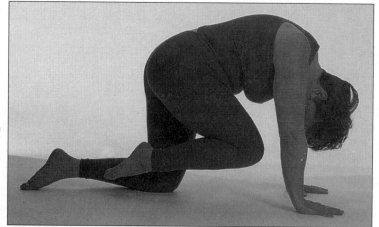

Figure 9-7:
The Cat Stretch with nose to knee.

10. **Repeat this action, extending your left leg back.**

    Beginners should practice one or two repetitions with each leg; more experienced students can practice three or four rounds.

11. **Sit back on your heels, and relax your torso onto your thighs; extend your arms by your sides, and rest your forehead on the floor, as illustrated in Figure 9-8.**

This posture is called the Folded Leaf, and it's a good resting posture.

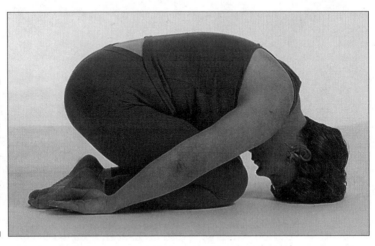

Figure 9-8:
The Folded
Leaf
position
allows your
muscles to
rest after
a good
stretch.

Chasing the wild Alley Cat

Alley cats tend to be a bit sassy and wild, and just as the Alley Cat's name implies, you have to try a bit harder to catch this cat. In this exercise, you begin with the Cat Stretch and if you're the type of person who likes to let your hair down now and then, you'll like this exercise.

The Alley Cat delivers all the benefits of the regular Cat Stretch, but it also gives your arms and shoulders an energizing stretch, and it promotes flexibility in your hips and thighs. (A soft exercise mat is an important prop for this exercise, to pad your knees from the floor and increases your stability.)

This exercise is definitely for those with healthy lower backs.

These steps help you tame the Alley Cat:

1. **Follow Steps 1 through 3 for the Cat Stretch; as you complete Step 3, you are on your hands and knees, with your back arched, and your head and hips tucked down (refer to Figure 9-4).**

2. **Inhale, and open your chest, by pulling your shoulders back, arching your back and expanding your chest as you lift your right arm up and out to the side of your torso.**

3. **Form a cat's claw with your hand, and mock the sound of an angry alley cat.**

Swipe your claws at the air a few times with all your wild cat sound effects.

4. **At the same time, lift and extend your left leg behind your back, keeping your knee bent (see Figure 9-9).**

Remember to make the sound of an angry cat.

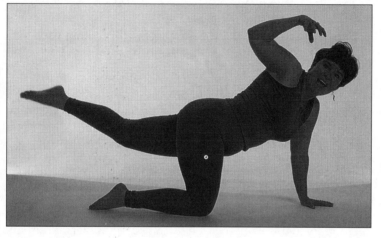

Figure 9-9:
Scratching and yowling like an Alley Cat is a fun and energizing part of this exercise.

5. **Reach behind your back with your left hand and grasp your right ankle.**

6. **Stretch your leg back and up as you hold this position for two complete breaths (see Figure 9-10).**

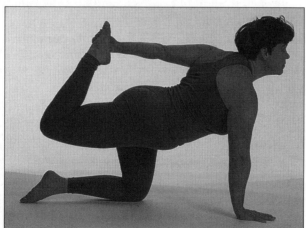

Figure 9-10:
This phase of the Alley Cat gives your torso, hips, and thighs an extra stretch.

7. On an inhalation, release and lower your leg, and then lower your back; let your back sway downward as you bend your arms to lower your chest and bring your chin to rest on the floor between your hands, gazing in front of you.

8. Exhale, and slowly draw your body up to return to the arched-back position you entered in Step 1.

9. Repeat Steps 2 through 8, using your right arm and left leg in Steps 4 and 5.

10. Finish by sitting back on your heels and relaxing your torso onto your thighs; extend your arms by your sides, and rest your forehead on the floor.

This is the Folded Leaf pose (refer to Figure 9-8).

Strengthening with push-ups

Power Cat Push-ups are quite a bit easier than traditional push-ups and have a yogic flavor. You practice traditional push-ups with legs straight, but Power Cat Push-ups let you rest on your knees, making it a "litter" easier.

Power Cat Push-ups work to strengthen your shoulders, arms, and pectoral muscles. This exercise is a great way to prepare you for the Power Yoga vinyasas. The core of Power Yoga are these flowing movements that keep your muscles working and your energy flowing between Yoga postures.

Use these steps to get the most out of your cat push-ups:

1. Form a "table" by supporting your body on your hands and knees, keeping your back straight but relaxed, and keeping your abdominal muscles firm to help support your back.

2. Move your arms forward about 6 inches, bend your elbows, interlace your fingers and on an exhalation, flatten your chin and entire torso down on to your extended hands (refer to Figure 9-5).

3. Inhale, and push your torso up to the arched-back cat position (refer to Figure 9-4).

4. Repeat this exercise 3–10 times, and relax into the Folded Leaf Posture (refer to Figure 9-8).

Standing Up, Warming Up

I don't want to forget the standing warm-ups, and you shouldn't either. Standing warm-ups are every bit as invigorating and useful as the "floor-based" models. Those I explain here help limber up your body to give you more freedom of movement and stability. And these warm-ups also help heat up your body's "engine" to keep it running strongly and smoothly.

Spinning with the Windmill

In the Windmill, you swing the upper part of your body, down, around, and up, moving in a circular motion like a windmill. You can get some real mental relaxation in this exercise if you imagine that you're a windmill turning softly in the breeze of a warm summer's day.

The Windmill helps to open the upper part of your body with gentle, flowing stretches. The spine is flexed and stimulated as you stretch the muscles of your back, stomach, and chest. This exercise brings a fresh supply of oxygenated blood to the brain, leaving you refreshed and invigorated.

Make like Don Quixote, and chase windmills using these steps:

1. **Begin the Windmill in a standing position, with your feet a little more than shoulder-width apart.**

2. **On an inhalation, raise your arms to reach up and over your head and expand your chest.**

3. **As you exhale, move your outstretched arms and torso down and to the left, in a circular motion.**

4. **On an inhalation, lift your arms and torso up and to the right, to complete the circle, as illustrated in Figure 9-11.**

   At the end of this exercise, you should end up where you started, with your arms stretched over your head.

5. **Repeat the steps, circling your arms and torso in the opposite direction, and performing two repetitions in each direction.**

   To get the most out of this exercise, make sure to time your movement with your breath.

Going into the Deep Lunge (Sirsangusthasana)

It's easy to see where this pose gets its name; in Sanskrit, *sirsa* means "head" and *angustha* relates to your big toe.

The Deep Lunge creates great strength in your legs and, at the same time, opens and expands your chest. This exercise also increases the mobility of your ankles and helps release tension from your neck. You'll notice that this posture gives you a sense of strength and self-confidence as your balance improves.

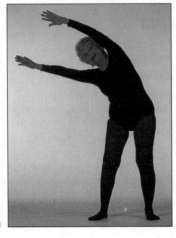

Figure 9-11:
The Windmill stretches your back, flexes your spine, and gets your blood pumping.

Lunge into this warm-up by following these steps:

1. **Start from a standing position, with legs firmly planted slightly more than shoulder-width apart.**

2. **Place your arms behind your back, interlock your fingers, and turn your left foot to the left.**

3. **Lift your arms up and behind you on an inhalation, expand your chest, and then exhale as you lunge down, lowering your face toward the toes of your left foot, as shown in Figure 9-12.**

   Try to keep you back straight, shoulders back and fingers interlaced and arms lifted off your back.

   Listen to your body. If this stretch is very painful, or just too much for you, you can just lower your nose toward your knee. This modification puts less strain on your back and legs.

4. **Hold this position for three complete breaths, and then lift up to the center on an inhalation.**

5. **Repeat these steps, lunging to the right.**

Expanding the toe touch

This exercise expands your chest, and stretches your arm and leg muscles. This simple warm-up is excellent for toning and strengthening your back, as well as warming up your body.

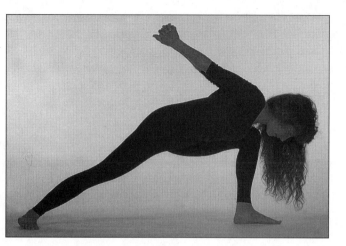

Figure 9-12:
The Deep Lunge stretches your back and legs.

Reach for your toes, not the stars, following these steps:

1. **Start this posture by standing up straight, with your shoulders back and your feet about four feet apart.**

2. **Turn your toes slightly inward and heels outward, grinding yourself into the earth.**

3. **Rest your arms by your sides, and relax.**

   This is known as the Expanded Mountain Pose.

4. **Bend your left elbow, and place your hand on your hip. Inhale as you lift your right arm up straight over your right shoulder.**

5. **Exhale, and lower your right arm, as you fold forward at your waist, trying to touch your left toes with your right hand.**

   If you aren't very flexible, bend your knees slightly. If you're more flexible, keep your legs straight.

6. **Inhale, and come to a standing position, as you lift your arm over your right shoulder and stretch toward the ceiling.**

7. **Repeat Steps 1 through 6 five times, and then lower your arms to your sides and return to the Expanded Mountain pose in Step1.**

8. **Repeat these steps, lifting your left arm and touching your right toe.**

Chapter 10

Saluting the Sun and Linking Your Poses

Since the dawn of Yoga practice, students have practiced the Sun Salutation in one form or another. The Sun Salutation is actually a *vinyasa* — a group of Yoga poses practiced in succession with fluid connecting movements. If you dissect the Sun Salutation you have various classical Yoga *asanas*.

In this chapter, I explain the ins and outs of practicing the Sun Salutations, and I give you a choice of three levels of Sun Salutations from which to choose. After you've fully powered up your solar-powered Yoga engine, I top off your tank by showing you five classic variations of Power Yoga *vinyasas* (linking movements). From *cool* or low-energy connecting links to the hottest of the hot, you discover the moves that make Power Yoga one of today's most popular fitness programs. So grab your shades, and get ready to turn up the heat.

Shedding Some Light on the Sun Salutation

The Sanskrit word for Sun Salutation is *suryanamaskar*. *Surya* means "sun" and *namaskar* is a "blessing, prayer, or salutation". Yoga's close ties to and appreciation for Nature certainly extend to this fundamental sequence. If not for the life-giving energy of our sun, life as we know it couldn't exist. The Sun Salutation is an important Yoga exercise and a healthy way to pay your respect to the sun — and to salute the ultimate good within each of us.

A Sun Salutation a day . . .

The Sun Salutation is a great way to begin and end your days.

Traditionally, Yoga practitioners have found that their energies are most powerful and calm during sunrise and sunset. Therefore, many yogis and yoginis practice the Sun Salutation during these times of day, using the tranquility of the environment during those hours to enhance the benefits of the exercise. Try it, and see whether you feel a new day dawning in your Power Yoga practice!

The Sun Salutation benefits literally your entire body. The stretching and counter-stretching of the torso rejuvenates your spine and helps relieve back pain. This exercise stretches and strengthens your arm and leg muscles and promotes flexibility in your ankle, knee, and hip joints. The gentle, fluid transition from stretch to counter-stretch, combined with Yoga breathing techniques, leaves your mind in a tranquil yet alert state. And these movements all turn up the energy in your own sun center located at the solar plexus. So, Sun Salutations rev up your metabolism.

Though all Sun Salutations share the same purpose and benefits, various forms of the exercise require different levels of energy. Soft-form and hard-form Sun Salutations exist. The hard-form Sun Salutations take a little more energy than the soft-form versions, and they let you create more heat and build more strength.

In this chapter, I divide the Sun Salutations into three categories in order to better accommodate students at any level of practice. Each category corresponds with a different type and energy level of salutation. Within each category, I dice things up a bit further by giving you a basic version and a "spicy" version that requires a bit more effort. You'll find these categories of Sun Salutation exercises:

✔ **Level 1 (Beginner) Energy Saver Sun Salutation:** The Energy Saver is a traditional Sun Salutation, derived from soft-form Yoga. This beginner Sun Salutation takes a minimal amount of energy. Regardless of your level of practice, you will find both the basic and the spicy versions of this Sun Salutation tranquil, fun, and beneficial.

✔ **Level 2 (Beginner to Intermediate) Feeling Your Oats Sun Salutation:** This mid-level Sun Salutation is derived from traditional, hard-form Yoga. This Sun Salutation takes a moderate amount of energy and generates more steam than the Energy Saver salutations. Both the basic and the spicy versions of the Feeling Your Oats Sun Salutation help you to build more strength and stamina for a progressive Power Yoga practice.

✔ **Level 3 (Intermediate to Advanced) Mother Lode Sun Salutation:** If you're feeling up to the challenge, you can take on the Mother Lode Sun Salutation. This salutation takes full power and generates enough heat and energy to melt the snow off your driveway. Both the basic and the spicy versions of the Mother Lode Sun Salutation help you to develop maximum strength and stamina.

Starting Up the Energy Saver

The Energy Saver is a good place to start if you're a beginning Power Yoga student. It requires minimum power and is suitable for Level 1 practitioners. Within this beginner category, I give you two choices of salutations:

✔ **Basic Energy Saver:** A classic soft-form Yoga Sun Salutation, this version requires a minimal amount of energy and is rated for the beginner.

✔ **Spicy Energy Saver:** Still a traditional soft-form Sun Salutation, this salutation is dressed up with a few extra moves to give it a bit more "heat" than the basic flavor. Even so, it remains a minimal-energy exercise.

Use your Yoga breathing technique with all Sun Salutations. For a refresher on the Yoga breathing techniques, see Chapter 7.

Beginning with the basic Energy Saver Salutation

The basic Energy Saver Salutation is the basis for many of the more elaborate Sun Salutations used in Yoga practice today. Follow these steps to perform the Energy Saver:

1. **Begin by standing straight, relaxed, and firmly grounded, with your feet together, spine straight, and shoulders back.**

2. **Extend your arms down by your sides, and direct your gaze forward, as illustrated in Figure 10-1a.**

   This is known as Mountain Pose I.

3. **Take a few slow, deep breaths to calm and relax your mind. On an inhalation, lift your arms slowly in front of your body and extend them over your head.**

   Keep your wrists loose, and synchronize your movement with your breathing.

4. **Arch slightly backward, and direct your gaze toward your hands, as shown in Figure 10-1b.**

   This posture is called the Mountain Pose II.

5. **Slowly bend your elbows, bring your palms together, and lower your hands to form a cross over your chest in prayer fashion, as you exhale and start into the Standing Forward Bend.**

6. **Continue your exhalation as you move further into your maximum Standing Forward Bend, placing your hands on the floor beside your feet, as shown in Figure 10-1c.**

   If you have trouble keeping your back straight in the Standing Forward Bend, keep your knees slightly bent.

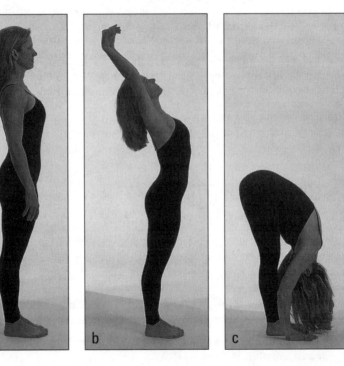

Figure 10-1: The first three steps of the basic Energy Saver Sun Salutation take you through Mountain Poses I (a) and II (b) and into the Standing Forward Bend (c).

a   b   c

7. **Take a large step backward with your right leg (your toes curled under) as you inhale, and let your knee rest on the floor.**

8. **Arch your torso upward as you gaze toward the sky.**

   Your hands are still on the floor on either side of your left foot; your left leg is bent at 90 degrees or more, and your right leg is extended behind you, as shown in Figure 10-2a. This is called the Runner's Stretch Posture.

9. **Exhale as you step back with your left leg to place it beside your right leg, behind you.**

10. **Lower your torso onto the floor.**

    Your hands are under your shoulders, your knees are slightly bent, your chest is resting on the floor, and your toes are pointed, as shown in Figure 10-2b. This is the Basic Four Limb Staff Pose.

    As you practice your Sun Salutation, try to create a fluid, continuous movement from one position to the next — like a slow dance. Ride the rhythm of your breath.

11. **Keep your knees slightly bent and resting on the floor, as you exhale all your air, lift your hips by pushing back with your arms and rest your hips on your heels. Lower your chest to the floor.**

    Your arms should be stretched out on the floor in front of you and your hips over your calf muscles, with your torso resting on your thighs, as you move into the Child's Pose, as shown in Figure 10-2c.

12. **On an inhalation, pull your torso forward with your arms and push down with your knees.**

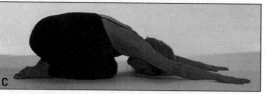
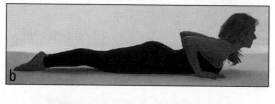

Figure 10-2: As you move from Runner's Stretch (a) through Basic Four Limb Staff (b) to Child's Pose (c), keep your movements as fluid as possible.

13. **Arch your body upward, moving into the Cobra Pose, as shown in Figure 10-3a.**

14. **Retrace your steps on an exhalation, as you lower your torso back down to the floor and pass through the Child's Pose (refer to Figure 10-2c).**

15. **Continue the exhalation as your lift your hips into the air, pushing your body up by straightening your legs and arms.**

    Your body forms a 90-degree angle from hips to hands and hips to feet as you move into the Downward Facing Dog Pose, as shown in Figure 10-3b.

16. **On an inhalation, bring your right leg forward between your hands.**

17. **Arch your torso upward as you gaze toward the sky, inhaling to expand your chest into Runner's Stretch.**

    Your hands are still by your sides as you fill your lungs with air. See Figure 10-2a.

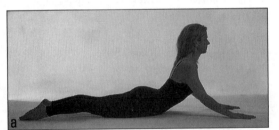

Figure 10-3:
Counter-
stretches
move from
Cobra Pose
(a) to
Downward
Facing Dog
(b) to
Runner's
Stretch.

18. **Bring your left foot forward, as you move back into the Standing Forward Bend (refer to Figure 10-1c) and exhale all your air.**

19. **On an inhalation, ripple your body slightly forward in a wavelike motion to come to a standing position; lift your arms in front of your body, keeping your wrists soft and relaxed.**

20. **With your hands extended over your head, arch your back softly.**

    See Figure 10-1b.

21. **Lower your arms to form a cross over your chest in prayer fashion as you exhale and return to the Mountain Pose I (refer to Figure 10-1a).**

22. **Repeat Steps 1 through 21 of this exercise, but begin with your left leg in Steps 7 and 16.**

Practice this Sun Salutation in groups of two, starting with two repetitions and working up to four.

Warming up to the spicy Energy Saver salutation

This Level 1 Sun Salutation adds a bit of spice to the basic version of the exercise by incorporating some extra moves. This sequence is another variation on a traditional soft-form Yoga salutation and is a good way for beginners to expand their salutation "repertoire" without taking on too much too soon.

1. **Begin by standing straight, relaxed, and firmly grounded, with your feet together, spine straight, and shoulders back.**

2. **Extend your arms down by your sides, and direct your gaze forward in Mountain I Pose (refer to Figure 10-1a).**

3. **Take a few slow, deep breaths to calm and relax your mind. On an inhalation, lift your arms slowly in front of your body and extend them over your head.**

   Keep your wrists loose, and synchronize your movement with your breathing.

4. **Arch slightly backward, and direct your gaze toward your hands in Mountain II Pose (refer to Figure 10-1b).**

   Join your movements into one continuous flow as you move from one position to the next in this salutation.

5. **Slowly bend your elbows, bring your palms together, and lower your hands to form a cross over your chest in prayer fashion, as you exhale and start into the Standing Forward Bend.**

6. **Continue your exhalation as you move further into your maximum Standing Forward Bend, placing your hands on the floor beside your feet (refer to Figure 10-1c).**

   If you have trouble keeping your back straight in the Standing Forward Bend, keep your knees slightly bent.

7. **Take a large step backward with your right leg as you inhale, and let your knee rest on the floor.**

   Your hands remain on the floor on either side of your left foot; your left leg is bent at 90 degrees or more, and your right leg is extended behind you (refer to Figure 10-2a).

8. **Arch your torso upward as you gaze toward the sky.**

9. **Expand your chest on an inhalation, lift your arms over your head, keeping your shoulders down, and touch your palms together with your arms fully extended and your gaze directed toward your hands.**

This is called the Kneeling Warrior I Pose, as illustrated in Figure 10-4.

As you lift your arms and torso upward, respect your own limits; don't try to lift your back further than is comfortable.

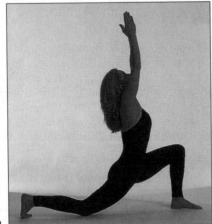

Figure 10-4:
Be sure that your point of gaze is directed toward your hands in the Kneeling Warrior I Pose.

10. **On an exhalation, lower your arms to form a cross over your chest, in prayer fashion, and return your hands to rest on the floor by your sides (refer to Figure 10-2a).**

11. **Continue the exhalation as you step back with your left leg, placing it beside your right leg behind you.**

12. **With your feet together, stiffen your body — with your arms and legs fully extended — like a solid plank or board.**

This is called the Plank Pose. Support your entire body with only your hands and feet, as if you were doing pushups. See Figure 10-5.

13. **Continue the exhalation as you lower your torso to the floor and drop your knees down.**

14. **Push your hips back over your calf muscles, and stretch your arms out on the floor in front of you in the Child's Pose (refer to Figure 10-2c).**

15. **On an inhalation, pull your torso forward with your arms and push with your feet.**

16. **Arch your torso upward into the Cobra Pose (refer to Figure 10-3a).**

When you move in and out of the Cobra Pose, uncoil slowly, like a snake, one vertebra at a time.

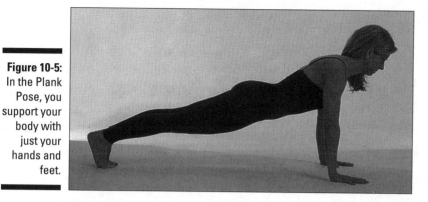

Figure 10-5:
In the Plank Pose, you support your body with just your hands and feet.

17. **Retrace your steps on an exhalation, as you lower your shoulders and torso back to the floor and pass through the Child's Pose (refer to Figure 10-2c).**

18. **Continue the exhalation as you lift your hips into the air by pushing down as you straighten your legs and arms.**

    Your body forms a 90-degree angle from hips to hands and hips to feet as you move into the Downward Facing Dog Pose (refer to Figure 10-3b). Hold this pose for two slow, deep breaths.

19. **On an inhalation, bring your right leg forward between your hands as you lower your left knee to the floor.**

20. **Arch your torso upward as you gaze toward the sky, inhaling to expand your chest and lifting your arms over your head in the Kneeling Warrior I Pose (refer to Figure 10-4, which shows the left leg forward).**

21. **On an exhalation, lower your arms to form a cross over your chest, in prayer fashion, and return your hands to rest beside your right leg in the Runner's Stretch Position (refer to Figure 10-2a).**

22. **Continue the exhalation, and bring your left leg forward to return to the Standing Forward Bend, as you exhale completely (refer to Figure 10-1c).**

23. **Return to a standing position on an inhalation as you ripple your body slightly forward in a wavelike motion.**

24. **Lift your arms in front of your body, and return to a standing arched position, with your arms over your head in the Mountain Pose II (refer to Figure 10-1b).**

25. **Lower your arms to form a cross over your chest, in prayer fashion, as you exhale and return to the Mountain Pose I (refer to Figure 10-1a).**

26. **Repeat Steps 1 through 25, but begin with your left leg in Step 7.**

Practice this Sun Salutation in groups of two, starting with two repetitions and working up to four.

Feeling Your Oats Sun Salutation

This intermediate, level 2 Sun Salutation has its roots in traditional hard-form Yoga, so it's right at home in your Power Yoga routine. In this section, I give the instructions for two versions of this intermediate exercise:

- **Basic Feeling Your Oats:** This salutation requires a moderate amount of energy and is appropriate for beginning- to intermediate-level students.

- **Spicy Feeling Your Oats:** This salutation adds a few extra moves to the basic version and requires more energy. This salutation is good for intermediate-level students.

Because the Feeling Your Oats salutation is hard-form Power Yoga, be prepared to exert a little more energy than in the Level 1 exercises. If you're a beginning-level student, practice the basic Feeling Your Oats salutation until you're comfortable with it; then move into the spicy version as your Yoga skills progress. Don't push it, and you'll have a great time with these intermediate-level exercises.

Getting comfortable with the Basic Feeling Your Oats Salutation

Power Yoga is popular today because people appreciate its high-energy workout. That same appreciation for "feeling the burn" has drawn people to this intermediate-level Feeling Your Oats version of the Sun Salutation. You'll also find that this salutation is a great training exercise for the *vinyasas* you use throughout your Power Yoga routines.

Seeking the energy of the sun

Aside from being a healthy exercise, the Sun Salutation is a demonstration of respect for the sun and its life-giving energy. Without this energy, life as we know it couldn't exist on Earth. The Sun Salutation, with its stretching, strengthening, and breathing exercises combined in peaceful, flowing movements, has a powerful effect on your body. It provides a soothing touch for your mind and body.

Follow these steps to perform the basic Feeling Your Oats salutation:

1. **Being in the Mountain Pose I (refer to Figure 10-1a), with your feet together, spine straight, and shoulders back.**

2. **Place your arms by your sides and gaze forward, standing up straight and solid, yet relaxed.**

3. **Lift your arms to your sides as you inhale and expand your chest; continue lifting your arms all the way up over your head, touch your palms together, and gaze up at your hands.**

   This is the Mountain Pose III, as shown in Figure 10-6.

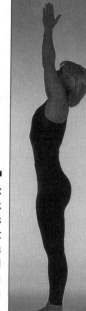

Figure 10-6:
Your back
remains
straight, but
retains its
natural
curves, in
Mountain
Pose III.

4. **On an exhalation, bend forward, keep your chest open, and lower your arms to your sides and down to the floor beside your feet as you enter the Standing Forward Bend.**

   Try to keep your back straight; if you're a beginner, keep your knees slightly bent to avoid rounding your lower back.

   You should now have reached your maximum stretch in the Standing Forward Bend position, with your legs straight.

5. **Place your hands on the floor, slightly in front of your feet; bend your knees if necessary (see Figure 10-1c).**

6. **Keeping your hands on the floor, arch your back and expand your chest as you inhale and look upward.**

   This posture, shown in Figure 10-7, is called the Jackknife Posture *(padangasana)*.

Figure 10-7: The Jackknife Posture, like the Jackknife swimmer's dive, folds your body in the middle to bring hands and toes together.

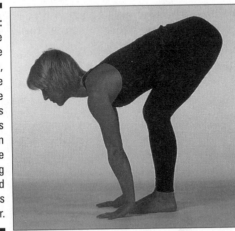

7. **Bend your knees as you step both legs back — one at a time — into a pushup position, with your body firm and solid, like a plank or board (refer to Figure 10-5).**

8. **Supporting your body with your hands and the toes of your flexed feet, exhale and lower your body until it's about one inch above the floor.**

   This is called the Four Limb Staff Position (see Figure 10-8). If supporting your body this way is too difficult, rest your torso on the floor, with your knees slightly bent in the Basic Four Limb Staff Position (refer to Figure 10-2b).

   As you lower you body from the Plank Pose to the Four Limb Staff, engage all your abdominal muscles and hold your Mula Bandha and Uddiyana Bandha muscle locks. (If you need a refresher on engaging your bandhas, see Chapter 7. For the location of the bandhas, check out the Cheat Sheet.)

9. **Pull your torso forward with your arms, and push up with your feet on an inhalation.**

10. **Arch your body up, push forward, and roll up onto the tops of your feet as you lift your torso upward.**

Figure 10-8:
The full Four
Limb Staff
Position,
*Chaturanga
Dandasana*
in Sanskrit.

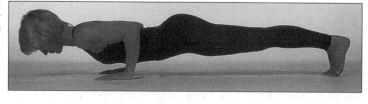

11. **Expand your chest, open your shoulders, and direct your gaze up toward the sky.**

    This posture is known as the Upward Facing Dog (see the Cheat Sheet at the front of the book).

    Initially, you may find the Upward Facing Dog to be much easier if you place a small pillow under your upper thighs, to take the pressure off your lower back. And, if you really want to get into the spirit of the Upward Facing Dog, imagine that you're a coyote and you just woke up from a nap. Give your body a stretch, and howl at the moon. Give it a try right now — I can't hear you!

12. **Exhale, lift your hips up into the air as you drop your head and shoulders down. Try to keep your arms straight and roll up on to the balls of your feet, with toes curled under, into the Downward Facing Dog.**

    If you feel pain or too much discomfort in the Downward Facing Dog Pose as you try to lower your heels to the floor, don't keep trying to push them down. Walk your feet up closer to your hands and bend your knees slightly, then try lowering your heels again. Alternatively, you can place a rolled towel under your heels for support.

13. **Hold the Downward Facing Dog Position (see the Cheat Sheet) for three complete breaths, and then step your feet, one at a time, back up between your hands, on an inhalation; continue inhaling as you arch your torso upward and expand your chest to return to the Jackknife Position that you reached in Step 6 (refer to Figure 10-7).**

14. **Drop your head forward, flatten your back, and return to your Standing Forward Bend as you exhale completely.**

15. **Raise your arms out to your sides as you expand your chest by inhaling.**

16. **Return to a standing position, lift your arms all the way up over your head, touch your palms together, and gaze toward your hands as you return to Mountain Pose III (refer to Figure 10-6).**

17. **Lower your arms softly to your sides as you exhale and return to Mountain Pose I.**

18. **Repeat this exercise three times.**

Moving up to the spicy Feeling Your Oats Salutation

The spicy Feeling Your Oats salutation requires moderate power and is really best suited for intermediate-level students. In this version of the Feeling Your Oats salutation, you jump back rather than step back during the movement between the Standing Forward Bend and the Plank Pose, and you extend the length of time you spend in the Downward Facing Dog Posture by adding breaths and some extended leg movements.

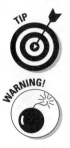

This Sun Salutation features lots of jumping in and out of different positions, so try to maintain a soft, fluid Yoga feel throughout these movements. Stay strong, yet relaxed and in control, as you flow from one position to the next.

If you have back problems, step rather than jump into poses. Any hard landing puts stress on your lower back.

Follow these steps to spice up the Feelings Your Oats Salutation:

1. **Begin in the Mountain I Pose, with your feet together, spine straight, and shoulders back.**

2. **Extend your arms down by your sides, and keep your gaze forward.**

   This stance should be solid but relaxed.

3. **Lift your arms out to the sides of your body as you inhale and expand your chest; continue lifting your arms all the way up over your head, touch your palms together, and direct your gaze toward your hands.**

4. **Bend forward on an exhalation, as you keep your chest open and lower your arms to your sides and down to the floor, placing your hands beside your feet.**

   Bend your knees if necessary to keep your back straight.

5. **Arch your back, expand your chest by inhaling, and look upward, keeping your hands on the floor.**

6. **Bend your knees, and jump both legs back, landing into a pushup position with your body firm and solid in the Plank Position (refer to Figure 10-5).**

7. **Exhale and lower your body to the floor, moving into the Four Limb Staff Position (refer to Figure 10-8).**

When you're jumping from the Standing Forward Bend to the Plank Pose, shift your weight forward, bend your elbows, and lean your shoulders out over your hands.

8. **Pull your torso forward with your arms, as you push forward with your feet on an inhalation.**

9. **Arch your body upward as you move into the Upward Facing Dog Pose.**

10. **Push forward, roll up onto the tops of your feet, lift your torso upward, and expand your chest and shoulders as you gaze upward.**

11. **Lift your hips into the air as you drop your head and shoulders on an exhalation, moving into the Downward Facing Dog Pose (refer to Figure 10-3b).**

12. **Spread your fingers, roll your shoulders outward, and lift your hips into the air.**

Your arms and legs should be fully extended, your chest open, and your gaze directed toward your toes.

13. **With your feet about 12 inches apart, try to lower your heels to the floor.**

As in the basic Feeling Your Oats salutation, don't try to push your heels to the floor if it causes you pain or discomfort. Instead, walk your feet closer to your hands, bend your knees slightly, and then try lowering your heels again; alternatively, place a rolled towel under your heels for support.

14. **Hold the Downward Facing Dog Position for five complete breaths, and then raise your right leg back and up, as high as you can, on an inhalation; try to keep your knee as straight as you can then lower it back to the floor on an exhalation.**

15. **Repeat these steps, but lift and lower your left leg this time.**

16. **Jump or step your feet back up between your hands on an inhalation; when both feet are between your hands, bend your knees and exhale.**

17. **With your hands on the floor, arch your torso upward on an inhalation as you expand your chest and arch your back; direct your gaze upward, as in the Jackknife Pose.**

18. **Return to the Standing Forward Bend, and exhale completely.**

19. **Lift your arms out to your sides as you expand your chest on an inhalation; return to standing with your back straight as you lift your arms all the way up over your head, palms touching and eyes gazing toward your hands in Mountain Pose III.**

20. **Lower your arms softly back by your sides as you exhale and return to the Mountain Pose I.**

    Repeat this exercise 3–5 times.

The Mother Lode Salutation

This is an intermediate- to advanced-level Sun Salutation, derived from a traditional hard-form style of Power Yoga. This Level 3 Sun Salutation requires lots of energy, but it offers big payoffs in increased strength, flexibility, and coordination. As with other exercises in this chapter, I give you two versions of the Mother Lode:

- ✔ **Basic Mother Lode:** A traditional hard-form style Sun Salutation, this version is suitable for intermediate to advanced students. Make sure that you're comfortable with this version of the Mother Lode before you move on to the spicy version.

- ✔ **Spicy Mother Lode:** This is a full-power Sun Salutation with a few more moves than the basic version. This baby lets you cut loose and go for the gold. It requires lots of energy and endurance, and it's suitable for intermediate to advanced students. When you run through this exercise, expect to hear your inner-Captain Kirk calling "Give me full power, Scotty!"

Mastering the basic Mother Lode Salutation

This Level 3 salutation is a good "step up" exercise for intermediate students. After you've become comfortable with this salutation, you should be ready to take on the hotter version in this section.

Use these steps to bring home the Mother Lode:

1. **Begin in the Mountain Pose I, with your feet together, spine straight, and shoulders back.**

2. **Extend your arms down by your sides as you gaze forward in a solid, yet relaxed stance.**

3. **Lift your arms out from the sides of your body as you inhale and expand your chest; continue lifting your arms all the way up over your head, bringing your palms together, and gazing at your hands.**

4. **Bend your knees, as if you were sitting in an imaginary chair.**

   This is the Powerful Chair Posture, as illustrated in Figure 10-9.

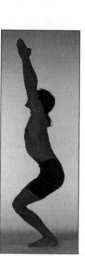

Figure 10-9:
When you move into the Powerful Chair Posture, keep your lower back flat, tuck your hips under, and gaze up toward your hands.

5. **On an exhalation, bend forward and keep your chest open as you move into a Standing Forward Bend (refer to Figure 10-1c).**

6. **Keep your hands on the floor, and inhale as you arch your back and expand your chest; direct your gaze upward.**

7. **Bend your knees, and jump both legs back, landing with your body firm and solid in the Plank Position (refer to Figure 10-5).**

8. **Exhale, and lower your body to the floor as you move into the Four Limb Staff (refer to Figure 10-8).**

9. **On an inhalation, pull your torso forward with your arms and push forward with your feet.**

10. **Arch your body upward into the Upward Facing Dog Pose.**

11. **Push forward, rolling up onto the tops of your feet, lifting your torso upward, expanding your chest, and opening your shoulders as you gaze upward.**

12. **Lift your hips into the air as you drop your head and shoulders on an exhalation, moving into the Downward Facing Dog Pose (refer to Figure 10-3b).**

13. **Spread your fingers, roll your shoulders outward, and lift your hips into the air.**

    Your arms and legs should be fully extended, your chest open, and your gaze directed toward your toes.

14. **With your feet about 12 inches apart, try to lower your heels to the floor.**

    Walk your feet in toward your hands and bend your knees slightly if you have trouble lowering your heels to the floor.

15. **On an inhalation, turn your left foot in sideways, rotating on the ball of your foot by bringing your heel in toward your right foot.**

16. **Take a large step forward with your right foot, so that your knee is positioned over your ankle and your thigh is parallel to the floor.**

17. **Expand your chest as you lift your arms out to your sides and up over your head; touch your palms together, and gaze upward as you move into the Full Warrior I Pose as shown in Figure 10-10.**

    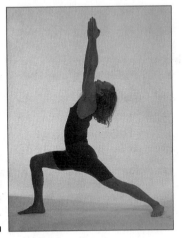

    To perform the classic Full Warrior I pose, you move into the full position in one inhalation. When you're mastering this pose, however, take extra breaths if you feel the need.

Figure 10-10: The Full Warrior I Pose stretches and strengthens your arms and legs.

18. **On an exhalation, lower your arms to your sides, and then lower your body to the floor as you step your right leg back behind you, and lengthen your body into the pushup position.**

19. **Continue to exhale as you lower your body into the Four Limb Staff Position (refer to Figure 10-8).**

20. **Pull your torso forward and arch your body into the Upward Facing Dog Pose.**

21. **Push forward, rolling up onto the tops of your feet, lifting your torso upward, and expanding your chest and shoulders as you gaze upward.**

22. **Lift your hips into the air as you drop your head and shoulders down on an exhalation, moving into the Downward Facing Dog Pose (refer to Figure 10-3b).**

23. **Spread your fingers, roll your shoulders outward, and lift your hips into the air.**

    Your arms and legs should be fully extended, your chest open, and your gaze directed toward your toes.

24. **With your feet about 12 inches apart, try to lower your heels to the floor.**

25. **Repeat Steps 15, 16, and 17 on the opposite side (and refer to Figure 10-10).**

26. **On an exhalation, lower your extended arms to your sides and back to the floor as you step your left leg behind you, lengthening your body into the Plank Pose; continue the exhalation as you lower your body into the Four Limb Staff.**

27. **Pull your torso forward again into the Upward Facing Dog Pose.**

28. **Lift your hips, and drop your head and shoulders again as you enter the Downward Facing Dog Pose.**

    As you hold the Downward Facing Dog Pose, keep your mind calm and relaxed, yet alert. If you have a weak wrist, elevate your palms one or two inches up off the floor with a rolled towel or a small book. You can also try a wedge made for just that purpose.

29. **Hold the Downward Facing Dog Position for three complete breaths, making sure to engage your Mula Bandha and Uddiyana Bandha muscle locks as you practice slow, deep Yoga breathing.**

30. **On an inhalation, jump your feet up between your hands.**

31. **With your hands on the floor, arch your torso upward and continue the inhalation as you expand your chest, arch your back, and gaze upward.**

32. **Return to the Standing Forward Bend, and exhale completely.**

33. **Lift your arms out to your sides as you inhale to expand your chest, and bend your knees as if you were sitting in a chair (refer to Figure 10-9 for the Powerful Chair Posture).**

34. **Return to a standing position, lifting your arms all the way up over your head, palms touching and eyes gazing toward your hands.**

35. **Lower your arms softly to your sides as you exhale, straighten your legs, and return to the Mountain Pose I (refer to Figure 10-1a).**

The ultimate workout in Yoga fitness

If you want to really spice things up and get the ultimate workout during your Sun Salutations, try your workout wearing wrist and ankle weights. Start with the lightest ones you can find, strap the weights on your wrist and ankles, and do your Sun Salutations very slowly. This truly is a workout, so I don't recommend it if you're an absolute beginner or still a bit out of shape. But as your fitness builds, you can use wrist and ankle weights to help improve your progress.

Heating up with the spicy Mother Lode Salutation

The spicy Mother Lode is a full-power version of the basic Mother Lode Salutation and a great addition to any late intermediate to advanced Power Yoga routine.

To perform the spicy Mother Lode Sun Salutation, repeat all the steps for the basic version, but hold the Downward Facing Dog poses for five complete breaths. Repeat all steps of this Sun Salutation five times.

Linking Your Power with Vinyasas

You've probably already figured out that the Sun Salutation, in any form, is really a series of Yoga *asanas* connected with *vinyasa* movements. You've played around with some *vinyasas,* but now it's time to add some of the most common and basic *vinyasas* to your repertoire of Power Yoga moves.

One of my main goals as your Power Yoga instructor is to make sure you feel comfortable using a variety of *vinyasas* to connect your Yoga postures. *Vinyasas* are the heart and soul of Power Yoga, and they serve four main functions:

- ✔ To keep energy moving from one Power Yoga pose to the next and to give your Power Yoga practice a feeling of fluidity and beauty

- ✔ To create internal heat within your body, which gives you more flexibility and helps your body release toxins

✔ To help distribute *prana* (life-force energy) throughout your body

✔ To clear your energy field for new poses — sort of like wiping a chalkboard clean to allow for new information

In this section, I list five separate *vinyasas;* each has its own character and is appropriate for particular phases of your practice. Some *vinyasas* are designed to link the standing poses and others link the sitting poses. Some are hotter, or more active; others are cooler and less physically demanding. Plan on using the cooler *vinyasas* when you first begin practicing Power Yoga. As you become more experienced, you can incorporate the hotter *vinyasas* into your routines.

The Rolling Stone Vinyasa

To practice the Rolling Stone, compact your body and gently roll in and out of this link. Your body remains strong during the movement, which is why it resembles the rolling stone for which this *vinyasa* is named. You use this *vinyasa* to connect seated poses and as a good training exercise for the full-seated *vinyasa* I describe next (the UFO). The Rolling Stone builds strength, endurance, and stamina, and it stretches out muscles of your back, chest, legs, and arms.

Like those other Rolling Stones you've heard of (the chain-smoking, rock-god variety), this *vinyasa* is really c-o-o-l. It's a good *vinyasa* to use when you're getting your Power Yoga feet wet. Don't forget to engage your Mula Bandha and Uddiyana Bandha throughout this *vinyasa* (and all others, for that matter). If you need a refresher on using the muscle lock bandhas, see Chapter 7; the Cheat Sheet shows you where they're located.

Follow these steps to practice the Rolling Stone *Vinyasa:*

1. **Start in the Seated Angle Pose, sitting on the floor with your legs extended in front of your torso.**

2. **Place your arms by your sides, and practice correct posture, with your spine straight and shoulders back, as you engage your *Mula Bandha* and *Uddiyana Bandha*.**

   Remember to practice Yoga breathing, and use the sound to help focus your attention on your movements during this *vinyasa.* (See the Cheat Sheet for Yoga breathing exercises and location of the Bandhas.)

3. **Bend your knees, cross your legs, and take an inhalation as you roll forward, pushing up on your hands to lift your hips; rest on your hands with your knees bent under your torso (see Figure 10-11a).**

4. **Use your legs to jump or step backward into the Four Limb Staff Position, supporting your body with your hands and the toes of your flexed feet; exhale and lower your body until it's about one inch above and parallel to the floor (see Figure 10-11b).**

   If this position becomes too difficult, rest your torso on the floor.

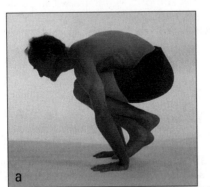

Figure 10-11:
Use the
Rolling
Stone
Vinyasa as a
connecting
link for
seated
postures.

a

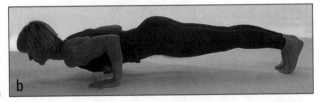

b

5. **On an inhalation, lift your torso into the Upward Facing Dog Posture.**

   Your torso should be arched and your chest expanded as you direct your gaze toward the sky (see Figure 10-12).

6. **On an exhalation, drop your head and lift your hips into the air.**

   You are now in the Downward Facing Dog Position (refer to Figure 10-3b).

7. **Bend your knees as you lift your head and look up beyond your hands; on an inhalation, walk or jump your legs up between your hands.**

8. **Support yourself with your hands as you softly lower your hips to the floor.**

9. **Straighten your legs up between your hands, and rest your arms at your sides in the Seated Angle Pose; exhale and relax.**

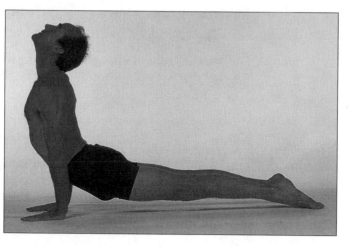

Figure 10-12:
The Upward Facing Dog is a central movement in the Rolling Stone *Vinyasa.*

The UFO Vinyasa

The UFO is a full-power version of the Rolling Stone *Vinyasa.* When you master this *vinyasa,* you'll lift up and float back and forth through your *vinyasa* like a UFO — "unidentified flying object" or "unbelievably funky object," whichever translation you prefer.

Though the UFO is also used to connect seated poses, it's a much hotter *vinyasa* than the Rolling Stone. If you're new to Power Yoga, I recommend that you master the Rolling Stone before you tackle this one. While doing the UFO, you generate lots of energy, but you remain calm and relaxed. This *vinyasa* offers the same types of benefits that you get from the Rolling Stone, but because it demands more, it delivers those benefits in larger quantities.

Follow these steps to practice the UFO *Vinyasa:*

1. **Follow Steps 1 through 3 for the Rolling Stone *Vinyasa,* except lift your hips and feet of the floor in Step 3.**

2. **Bend your legs and inhale as you lift your torso off the floor and pivot your hips; glide your legs back into a smooth landing in the Plank Position (refer to Figure 10-5).**

   If you need a boost during your "jump through," use a pair of Yoga blocks as props under your hands.

3. **On an inhalation, lift your torso into the Upward Facing Dog Posture, with your torso arched, your chest expanded, and your gaze directed toward the sky (refer to Figure 10-12).**

4. **On an exhalation, drop your head and lift your hips into the air.**

   You are now in the Downward Facing Dog Position (refer to Figure 10-3b).

5. **Lift your torso as you glide your legs in for a safe landing between your hands — into Seated Angle Pose shown in Figure 10-13.**

6. **Exhale and relax.**

The Missing Link Upward Vinyasa

No, this *vinyasa* doesn't require that you learn to walk like Sasquatch! I developed (and named) this *vinyasa* because traditional Yoga didn't offer a movement to connect seated poses to standing poses. This is a great *vinyasa* (if I do say so myself), and it's perfectly appropriate for both rookies and experienced Power Yoga practitioners.

In the Missing Link, you stretch and counter-stretch your back and neck, and you invigorate your spine with the movement's wavelike motion. This *vinyasa* teaches balance, grace, and self-confidence. The brain receives a gentle, peaceful vibration from the *vinyasa's* fluid movement and quiet transition. This cooler *vinyasa* requires minimum amounts of energy and is poetry in motion.

Follow these steps to practice the Missing Link *Vinyasa:*

1. **Start this *vinyasa* from the Seated Angle Pose as shown in Figure 10-13. Engage your Mula Bandha and Uddiyana Bandha now (see the Cheat Sheet).**

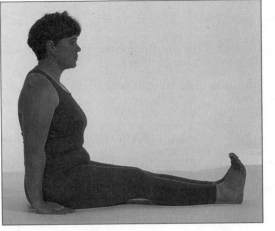

Figure 10-13:
The Seated Angle Pose is a basic Yoga — and Power Yoga — posture.

Training tips for accomplishing the UFO Vinyasa

Remember when you were a kid and used training wheels on your bike? You're still just a kid at heart, so I want to give you some training wheels for your *vinyasas.* To help with your otherworldly floating in the UFO, place your hands on Yoga blocks during the "jump through" between the Four Limb Staff and the Plank Positions. The blocks give you some extra clearance during this movement, and they help work your pectoral, upper arm, and stomach muscles. Make sure you're using strong, good-quality blocks that can support your body and give you at least a four-inch boost. Over time, you can use increasingly smaller blocks until you don't need them anymore.

2. Exhale completely, and then inhale as you expand your chest and lift your arms out to your sides and over your head (see Figure 10-14a).

3. On an exhalation, slowly bend your elbows as you fold your arms over your chest in prayer fashion.

4. As you lower your arms, bend your knees and bring your feet in toward your torso.

5. With your knees drawn up to your hands, separate your hands and lower your arms to your sides (see Figure 10-14b).

You should now be sitting in a compact ball, with your knees tucked into your body, your arms down by your sides, and your hands resting on the floor. This is called the Beach Ball Pose.

Figure 10-14:
The Missing Link *vinyasa* takes you from a seated pose (a) through the Beach Ball Pose (b), and eventually to a standing posture.

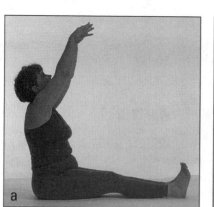
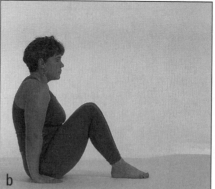

6. **Still exhaling, push against your hands to raise your hips from the floor as you roll your torso forward and drop your head, placing your weight on your feet; flow into a Standing Forward Bend (see Figure 10-15).**

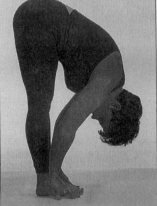

Figure 10-15: The Standing Forward Bend is a popular transition pose.

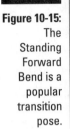

Steps 4, 5, and 6 should all be done in one exhalation, but if you can't quite handle that yet, take extra breaths as necessary. As your Power Yoga skills build, so will your ability to match your breathing to the ideal in this posture.

7. **Expand your chest as you lift your arms out to the sides of your torso and up over your head, and come to a full standing position.**

Your body should form a straight line now, with your arms stretched straight over your head and your eyes gazing toward your hands (refer to Figure 10-1b).

8. **Stand up straight, as you lower your arms toward your sides and gaze forward in the Mountain I Pose (refer to Figure 10-1a).**

The Monkey Jump Vinyasa

When you practice this *vinyasa,* you look like a monkey jumping into a wide, playful stance. Both beginning and more advanced Power Yoga students use this *vinyasa.* The Monkey Jump maintains moderate body heat and keeps your energy flowing as you move between many of the standing *asanas.*

The Monkey Jump strengthens your ankles and leg muscles and teaches you to combine softness with power in your Power Yoga workouts. This *vinyasa* also can improve your balance, rhythm, and coordination, and over time, it can open up tight shoulders and help relieve tension.

Follow these steps to practice the Monkey Jump *Vinyasa:*

1. **Start this *vinyasa* from the Mountain I Pose: standing with good posture — spine straight and shoulders back (refer to Figure 10-1a).**

2. **Keep your feet together and your arms by your sides, and take a few slow, complete breaths; relax.**

3. **On an inhalation, lift your arms over your head, with your palms facing outward and your wrists loose and relaxed; try to make yourself look like a monkey raising your loose, relaxed arms, as in Figure 10-16.**

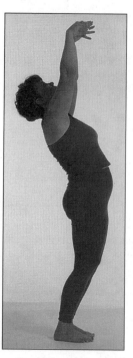

Figure 10-16:
Part of the
Monkey
Jump
involves
raising your
loose,
monkey-like
arms.

4. **On an exhalation, lower your arms and cross them in front of your body; at the same time, bend your knees as if you were preparing to jump (see Figure 10-17a).**

5. **As you start an inhalation, jump, throwing your arms out and upward and spreading your feet about one foot apart (see Figure 10-17b).**

6. **As you land, bend your knees deeply to absorb the shock; bring your arms over your head, with palms facing outward and elbows bent (see Figure 10-17c).**

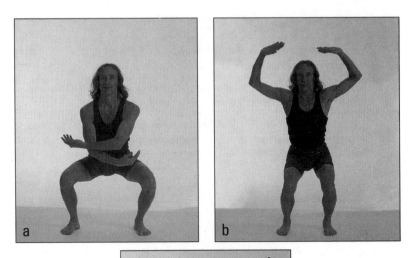

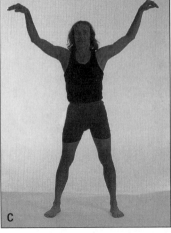

Figure 10-17:
The Monkey Jump earns its name as you crouch, jump, then land with your legs bent to absorb the shock.

7. **When you land, start your exhalation and straighten your legs as you lower your arms to your sides into Expanded Mountain Pose, shown in Figure 10-18.**

8. **To get back to the center, do the same jump in reverse; follow Steps 3 through 7, jumping your feet back together again.**

If the Monkey Jump *Vinyasa* feels awkward and uncomfortable to you, don't give up on it — just try some variations. Instead of jumping your feet apart, try stepping them apart. After you've mastered the Monkey Jump this way, you can move up to the full-jump version.

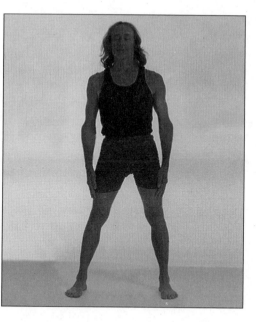

Figure 10-18:
Exhale and lower your arms into the Expanded Mountain Pose as you land in the Monkey Jump.

The Monkey Swings on Vines Vinyasa

After you know how to jump like a monkey, why not try swinging on some vines? In the Monkey Swings on Vines *Vinyasa,* you practice some broad, sweeping movements as you jump into the "vines" of this powerful, full-energy *vinyasa.* But no matter how much you swing, don't forget to stay relaxed and calm and keep your movements fluid and controlled.

The Monkey Swings on Vines strengthens your legs, ankles, and knees as it teaches you balance and coordination. The jump in this *vinyasa* is larger than the jump in the Monkey Jump, so this *vinyasa* calls for some extra energy, rhythm, and coordination.

Follow these steps to practice the Monkey Swings on Vines *Vinyasa:*

1. **Follow Steps 1 through 4 for the Monkey Jump.**

2. **Throw your arms up — keeping them very relaxed and loose like a monkey — as you jump up into the air and make a half turn to the right. Land with your feet slightly more than a shoulder's width apart.**

   Keep your knees flexed to absorb the shock of your landing (see Figure 10-17b).

   Your arms should still be over your head, elbows slightly bent, palms facing outward, and wrists relaxed.

3. **As you straighten your knees, lower your arms to your sides and relax in the Expanded Mountain Pose (refer to Figure 10-18).**

If you're a rookie Power yogi or yogini, you may want to step to the right, instead of jumping, when you're first learning this *vinyasa*. The stepping movement is smoother for beginners; just imagine yourself swinging on vines as you take a really wide step to the right.

4. **To get yourself back to the center, exhale as you lower your arms and cross them in front of your body, and bend your knees as if you were preparing to jump for those vines.**

5. **Now inhale as you jump, lifting you arms over your head and taking the half turn back to the left.**

6. **Land with your feet together, your knees bent, and your arms over your head; exhale as you straighten your legs and lower your arms to your sides.**

Congratulations, monkey — you did it!

Chapter 11

Taking a Walk in the Park: A Minimum Power Routine

1 named this routine Just a Walk in the Park because it's a fairly easy routine that makes a good introduction to Power Yoga. This workout is perfect if you have just under an hour for your practice. You can complete it in 30 to 45 minutes.

In this chapter, I give you some brief background information about the postures of this short, well-balanced workout, and I show you just when to incorporate a linking movement, or *vinyasa,* to move from one posture to the next. Because this routine takes relatively little time, you get a full dose of Power Yoga benefits in a small package — that's a good deal from all angles. So grab your Yoga mat, put on those Power Yoga togs, and get moving!

Talking before Walking

Just a Walk in the Park is the easiest Power Yoga routine in this book. It gives you a gentle introduction to a full Power Yoga workout. This routine leaves you feeling energized and refreshed, and I'm sure you'll enjoy it. To get the most from this walk, keep these tips in mind:

✔ **Prepare your space:** Make sure that your workout room is warm and has a good supply of fresh air. Have a good, soft Yoga mat ready, along with some pillows, towels, and blocks. (If you're a beginner or you have physical limitations, you may want to use Yoga props.)

✔ **Follow the instructions:** Doing as I say is the key to reaping the benefits of this routine.

✔ **Take your time:** If you rush just to get through this — or any — Power Yoga routine, you miss out on many of the mental and physical benefits.

✔ **Incorporate Yoga breathing techniques:** Keeping your breathing going is crucial during every phase of your workout.

One of the most important concepts in Power Yoga is to practice a routine that's appropriate for your present level of Yoga fitness. I say "Yoga fitness," rather than fitness in general, because even the most fit individuals can find the stretching and strengthening exercises of Power Yoga to be a challenge in the beginning. If you're out of shape, take it easy and move through this routine slowly and without putting undue strain on your muscles (or your good humor).

The Beginner's Routine: A Walk in the Park

This routine starts you off with some Power Yoga breathing techniques, moves you softly into a few warm-ups, and then gives you a mild *vinyasa* to take you to a standing pose. After you get a taste of some powerful standing poses, you move softly back to the floor and practice the traditional, whole-body finishing poses, or *asanas*. You complete your journey with breathing and deep relaxation. Table 11-1 gives you a quick overview of the Walk in the Park Power Yoga routine.

Table 11-1	Just a Walk in the Park Routine	
Exercise	*Duration*	*Reference*
Yoga breathing	5–10 breaths	Cheat Sheet
Neck and shoulders	As needed	"Working the kinks out . . ."
Cat Stretch	2 repetitions	Figures 9-4 to 9-7
Cat Pushups	3 repetitions	Figure 11-1
Downward Facing Dog	5 breaths	Cheat Sheet
Missing Link Upward	As needed	Figures 10-13–10-15; Figure 10-1b&a
Powerful Chair	5 breaths	Figure 10-9
Wall Pushups to Down Dog	5–10 repetitions	Figure 11-2; Cheat Sheet
Warrior I	5 breaths	Figure 11-3
Missing Link Downward	As needed	Figures 10-15–10-14, 10-13

Exercise	Duration	Reference
Seated Forward Bend	5 breaths	Figure 11-4
Boat	3 breaths	Figure 11-6
Cobra	3 repetitions	Figure 10-3a
Yoga breathing	5 breaths	Cheat Sheet
Deep relaxation	5–10 minutes	Figure 14-1

Starting well is breathing well

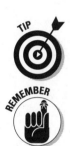

Always start your Power Yoga practice with Yoga breathing to find your center and quiet your mind. Check out the Cheat Sheet for a reminder of how to do this.

This exercise begins in the Easy Posture, but as you gain more experience in Power Yoga, you can substitute any of the seated positions in Chapter 8. In the course of this routine, you'll also use Yoga breathing, the seated postures, and the Jnana Mudra hand position featured in that chapter, so if you need a refresher on any of these techniques, Chapter 8 is the place to go before you begin this routine.

Follow these steps to begin your Walk in the Park:

1. **Sit cross-legged on the floor with your spine straight and your shoulders back.**

   If you find this uncomfortable, experiment with placing a small but firm pillow or rolled blanket under just the bony part of your seat (leave those cheeks behind!). If you still feel uncomfortable or if your knees just hang high in space, place a small supportive pillow under each thigh just above the knee.

   If you're a beginning Power Yoga student, you may find it more comfortable to sit on the edge of a small pillow or on the edge of a chair until you gain more flexibility.

2. **Extend your arms over your knees, resting your wrists on your knees, with your palms facing upward.**

3. **Form *Jnana Mudra* with your hands by bending your index finger in to touch the tip of your thumb; your remaining fingers should be straight, but not stiff or tense.**

4. **Practice your Yoga breathing (see the Cheat Sheet).**

Allow your breathing to calm your mind and body and help center your thoughts on your practice. Continue your Yoga breathing for 5–10 slow, deep breaths.

5. **Open your eyes, and go on to the neck and shoulder exercise listed in the next section.**

Working the kinks out of your shoulders and neck

The steps below walk you through these powerful neck and shoulder exercises. If you need more background information, refer to Chapter 9.

Follow these steps to warm up your neck and shoulders:

1. **Sit on the floor, with your spine straight and shoulders back; keep your arms relaxed and your hands resting in your lap.**

   If sitting on the floor is uncomfortable, sit on the edge of a heavy chair.

2. **On an inhalation, rotate your shoulders back as you lift them toward your ears; then, as you exhale, finish the backward rotation as you lower your shoulders to their original position.**

3. **Repeat Step 2, reversing the direction of your shoulder rotation.**

   Repeat each rotation three or four times, and then relax your shoulders.

4. **Maintain your erect, relaxed sitting position; on an exhalation, tilt your head forward and let your chin drop to your chest.**

   You'll feel the muscles in the back of your neck stretch.

5. **Inhale, and lift your head back to its upright position.**

6. **Exhale, and tilt your head back as far as you can without hurting anything.**

   You'll feel the muscles in the front of your neck and under your chin stretch.

7. **Inhale again, and lift the head back to the center.**

8. **Repeat Steps 4 through 7 four times, and then return to your original upright posture.**

9. **Exhale, and lower your head to your right shoulder; inhale, and raise your head to its original position.**

10. **Exhale, lower your head to the left side, and then go back to the center on an inhalation.**

11. **Relax for three complete breaths.**

    Use your Yoga breathing technique for maximum benefits.

12. **On an exhalation, turn your head to the right; keep your head level as you gaze over your right shoulder; inhale and turn your head back to look straight ahead.**

13. **Repeat Step 12, turning your head and gazing to the left on an exhalation, and back to the center on an inhalation.**

14. **Finish by closing your eyes and relaxing for three complete breaths.**

Moving into the Cat Stretch

The Cat Stretch is a wonderful warm-up exercise because it affects almost every part of your body. Chapter 9 covers the details of this posture, so if you need a refresher, you can refer to that chapter and to Figures 9-4–9-7.

Follow these steps to stretch like a cat:

1. **Start from a kneeling position; sit back on your heels, with your toes pointed backward.**

   Your back should be straight, and you should feel your neck lengthen.

2. **Lift your hips, and place your hands on the floor so that you're resting on your hands and knees.**

3. **Keep your back straight, but not rigid, and relax as you take three slow, deep breaths.**

   Have your hands right under your shoulders and your knees right under your hips — this is the Table Pose.

4. **On an exhalation, arch your back like a cat; relax your neck as you drop your head downward and gaze toward your knees.**

5. **On an inhalation, lower your back and let it sway downward as you bend your arms to lower your chest and bring your chin to rest on the floor between your hands.**

6. **Exhale, and slowly draw your body up and return to the arched-back position you reached in Step 4.**

   Time your moves with your breathing. Take your time, and try to flow from one position to the next.

7. **On an inhalation, sway your back downward again, but keep your arms straight and lift your head upward as you extend your right leg back and upward.**

   Your body should form a smile. Don't swing or jerk into this posture: Try to keep your movements fluid and soft as you lift your head and extend your leg back and up at the same time.

8. **On an exhalation, reverse the stretch by arching your back again, dropping your head, and bending your right knee toward your chest; try to touch your nose with your knee.**

9. **Repeat Steps 7 and 8, but extend your left leg this time.**

10. **Repeat these steps 2–4 times, and then relax into the Child's Pose (refer to Figure 10-2c).**

11. **Relax for two breaths, and then push your torso off the floor and come to rest on your hands and knees.**

Strengthening with Power Cat Push-Ups

The Power Cat Push-Ups strengthen the shoulder, arm, and pectoral muscles. This is a great exercise to prepare you for the UFO Power Yoga *vinyasa*.

Follow these steps to perform the Power Cat Pushups:

1. **Form a "table" by supporting your body on your hands and knees, with back straight but relaxed (see Figure 11-1a).**

   This is the Table Pose.

2. **Move your arms forward slightly, bend your elbows, and on an exhalation, lower your whole torso flat to the floor (see Figure 11-1b).**

   If you can't get all the way down at first, lower as far as you can and still push yourself up again. You'll soon be doing the full Power Cat Push-Up!

3. **Inhale, and push your torso up to the starting position on your hands and knees (as in Figure 11-1a again).**

4. **Repeat these steps 3–10 times, and then relax into the Folded Leaf (refer to Figure 9-8).**

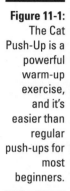

Figure 11-1:
The Cat Push-Up is a powerful warm-up exercise, and it's easier than regular push-ups for most beginners.

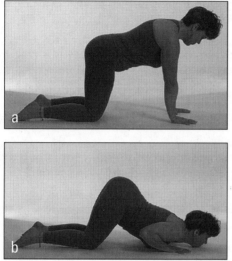

Stretching into the Downward Facing Dog (Adho Mukha Svanasana)

The phrase *adho mukha* (pronounced Ahd-ho Mook-ha) means "downward facing," and *svan* (pronounced shvahn) means "dog." The Downward Facing Dog Position resembles a dog stretching after awakening from his nap. As the dog awakens, he stretches his hips high in the air while he lengthens his entire spine and stretches his back. If you've ever been around a dog, you've seen this posture, and you may have thought "Oh, that looks like it feels so good."

Follow these steps to find out how good Fido feels when he stretches:

1. **Start from the Cat Prep Position: Rest on your hands and knees, with your hips, back, neck, and head forming a straight line.**

   Your knees should be directly under your hips and your hands directly under your shoulders.

2. **Roll up on your toes, and *slowly* straighten your legs to push your hips upward, and drop your head toward the ground; keep your arms straight and elbows relaxed.**

   Keep your shoulders wide and away from your ears, and your feet about a foot apart.

3. **Try to flatten your soles on the ground as your legs straighten; your feet should be about one foot apart.**

   If you can't comfortably straighten your legs, don't force it! Don't worry if you can't straighten your legs when you first try this posture. Power Yoga is supposed to feel good, so don't push too hard.

4. **Without straining or locking your elbows or knees, try to create a 90-degree angle with your body as you make a straight line from your heels to your hips and another straight line from your hips to your hands.**

5. **Gaze toward your toes, and begin taking slow breaths; try to hold this position for 3–5 complete breaths (see the Cheat Sheet).**

6. **Relax, lower your knees to the ground, and fold your body in half, so that your seat rests near your heels and your forehead reaches all the way to the floor.**

   Again, don't force yourself. Just relax.

7. **Stretch your arms in front of you, with palms facing downward.**

   Keeping a relaxed and extended neck and throat, get as close to the floor as you can. This is called the Extended Child's Pose.

8. **Remain in this position as you take a few slow, deep breaths, and then slowly lift your torso and return to sitting on your knees in preparation for the next exercise.**

Moving with the Missing Link Upward

This *vinyasa* is introduced in Chapter 10. This cool *vinyasa* keeps your energy flowing.

Follow these steps to achieve the Missing Link Upward:

1. **Start this *vinyasa* from the Seated Angle Pose, sitting on the floor with your legs stretched straight before you and your arms at your sides; engage your Mula Bandha and Uddiyana Bandha now (see the Cheat Sheet for the location of these muscle locks).**

2. **Exhale completely, and then inhale as you expand your chest and lift your arms out to your sides and over your head.**

3. **Start your exhalation, and slowly bend your elbows as you fold your arms over your chest in prayer fashion; as you fold your arms, bend your knees and bring your feet toward your torso.**

4. **When your knees are drawn up to your hands, separate your hands and lower your arms to your sides.**

   You should now be sitting in a compact ball, with your knees tucked into your body, your arms by your sides, and your hands resting on the floor.

5. **Still exhaling, push against your hands to raise your hips from the floor as you roll your torso forward and drop your head.**

   These movements help you flow into a Standing Forward Bend.

   Steps 3, 4, and 5 should all be done in one exhalation, but if you can't quite handle that yet, take extra breaths as necessary. As your Power Yoga skills build, so will your ability to match your breathing to the ideal in this posture.

6. **Expand your chest as you lift your arms out to your sides, and come to a full standing position; stretch your arms straight up over your head, and gaze up toward your hands.**

7. **Stand up straight as you lower your arms toward your sides and gaze forward in the Mountain Pose I.**

Building stability with the Powerful Chair (Utkatasana)

The Sanskrit word *Utkata* means "fierce or powerful." In this posture, you take on the characteristics of a strong and powerful chair. In the Powerful Chair Posture, you strengthen and firm the muscles of your legs, expand your chest, and release tension from your shoulders.

Follow these steps to achieve the Powerful Chair Pose:

1. **Stand up straight, with shoulders back, spine straight, and vision forward; keep your feet together, and stand strong, yet relaxed.**

2. **Start taking slow, deep inhalations and exhalations, and practice your Yoga breathing throughout this exercise.**

3. **On an inhalation, lift your arms out to your sides and over your head, bringing your palms together.**

4. **At the same time, bend your knees and come to a half sitting position, as if you were preparing to sit in a chair; gaze up toward your hands, and keep your lower back flat, tucking your tailbone forward. Feel your abdominal muscles engage (refer to Figure 10-9).**

5. **Hold this position for 5–10 slow, deep breaths.**

Strengthening your upper body with Wall Push-Ups and the Standing Dog Stretch

Wall Push-Ups strengthen the muscles of your arms and shoulders and give your upper-body muscles a great stretch. In this exercise, you do some modified push-ups against a wall, and you finish with a Standing Dog Stretch.

1. **Stand facing a wall, and extend your arms in front of you, toward the wall.**

   With your arms extended, your hands should be about 1–2 feet from the wall.

2. **From your standing position, lean forward and support yourself against the wall with your hands.**

3. **Exhale, and bend your arms to lower your chest to the wall; inhale and push yourself away from the wall by straightening your arms, as shown in Figure 11-2.**

4. **Repeat these steps 5–10 times.**

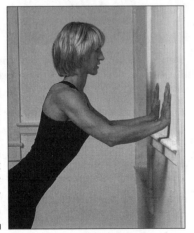

Figure 11-2: Move fluidly through your Wall Push-Ups, without jerking or locking your elbows.

To make your Wall Push-Ups more difficult, move out away from the wall; to make them easier, move closer to the wall.

5. **When you finish your push-ups, place your hands on the wall at about head level; keeping your arms straight, lean toward the wall, drop your head and shoulders downward, and extend your hips backward as if you were pushing a heavy load.**

This exercise, called The Dog Stretch, gives your shoulders a great stretch and releases tension.

6. **Relax and return to a standing position.**

Building balance with the Warrior 1 (Virabhadrasana)

The Sanskrit word *Virabhadra* means "Powerful hero warrior in Hindu legend." In Power Yoga, you use three variations of the Warrior Pose. In the Warrior I, used in this exercise, your arms come together pointed toward the sky.

The Warrior I Pose opens your chest and shoulders, and works to stimulate the nerves in your spine and to correct its alignment. This pose strengthens the muscles of your legs, opens your hips, and builds flexibility in your back and ankles. The Warrior I Posture improves your balance and can leave you feeling refreshed and confident.

Follow these steps to be a warrior, or at least feel like one:

1. **Start this posture from the Expanded Mountain Pose: Stand with your spine straight, shoulders back, arms at your sides, and feet about four feet apart (see Figure 11-3a).**

2. **Pivot on your feet to turn your body to the right until your right foot points straight to your right and your left foot is at a 45-degree angle from your right.**

   Your hips, shoulders, and torso should be squarely aligned to your right and your feet firmly planted on the ground.

3. **Lunge forward by bending your right knee until it forms a 90 degree angle from your hamstring to calf muscle.**

   Your knee should be over your heel and your thigh parallel to the floor.

4. **On an inhalation, lift your arms out to your sides and over your head, straighten your arms, touch your palms together, and point toward the sky.**

   Tilt your head back only as far as necessary to see your thumbs. Remember to keep your shoulders broad and down from your ears.

5. **Drop your head back and stretch your torso upward, as shown in Figure 11-3b, keeping your back foot flat on the floor.**

   If this is too difficult or uncomfortable, turn your toes downward on your left leg and rest on your toes.

Figure 11-3:
From the Expanded Mountain Pose (a), you pivot to the right, and then lower your body into the Warrior I Posture (b).

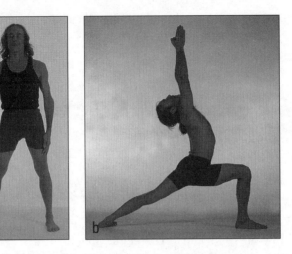

6. **Hold this position for 5–10 complete breaths, and then inhale and straighten your right leg.**

7. **Drop your arms to your sides, return to the Expanded Mountain Pose (as described in Step 1), and relax.**

8. **Repeat Steps 3 through 7, but lunge on your left leg this time.**

Finding the Missing Link Downward

It's time to take the Missing Link in the opposite direction to return you to the floor for your seated asanas.

Follow these steps to achieve the Missing Link Downward:

1. **Start from the Mountain I Pose: Stand up straight, with your shoulders back and your arms down by your sides (see Figure 10-1).**

2. **On an inhalation, lift your arms out to your sides and over your head, and touch your palms together in the Mountain III Pose as seen in Figure 10-16. (see the Cheat Sheet).**

3. **Exhale, and fold forward at your hips, moving into a Standing Forward Bend as you lower your arms toward your feet (refer to Figure 10-15).**

   Rest your hands on the floor beside your feet.

4. **Inhale, and bend your knees as if you were preparing to sit in a chair.**

5. **Lift your head upward, and continue lowering your body until your hips touch the floor; support your hips with your hands on the floor in the Beach Ball Pose, as shown in Figure 10-14b.**

6. **Exhale, and straighten your legs in front of you, resting into the Seated Angle Pose and forming a 90-degree angle from head to hips and hips to feet.**

Stretching your leg and back muscles with the Seated Forward Bend (Paschimottanasana)

The Sanskrit word *paschima* translates as "west." As you face the East, your back is to the West. This exercise stretches muscles on the back of your body — the back of your legs, the muscles along your spine, and your shoulders and upper back — and therefore is named for the direction that those muscles belong to.

Follow these steps to practice stretching your "west" side:

1. **Start from the Seated Angle Pose (see the Cheat Sheet). Exhale completely.**

2. **With an inhalation, lift your arms in front of your body and over your head; keep your wrists soft as you completely fill your lungs with air.**

3. **On an exhalation, gently lower your arms outward in a circular motion, reaching toward your toes, as shown in Figure 11-4a.**

4. **If you're relatively flexible, try to rest your torso on your thighs and take hold of your toes with your hands, keeping your feet flexed upward; relax and hold this position for five slow, deep breaths.**

This is the Extended Seated Forward Bend, as shown in Figure 11-4b.

Figure 11-4:
The Seated Forward Bend (a) and Expanded Seated Forward Bend (b) stretch the whole back of your body — neck to calves.

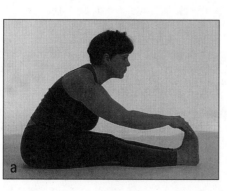
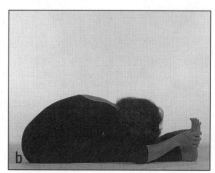

ALTERNATIVE

As an alternative, you can place a pillow under your knees for support and place your hands on your shins, instead of reaching for your toes. You can also wrap a Yoga strap around your feet and hold the ends of the strap, as shown in Figure 11-5, rather than grasping your feet in your hands.

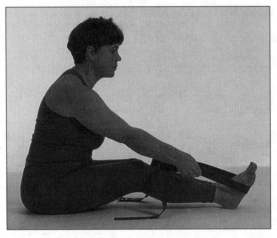

Figure 11-5:
A Yoga strap can help you get the same great stretch in the Seated Forward Bend with less strain on your back.

5. **On an inhalation, slowly return your torso to an upright position as you lift your arms over your head, keeping your wrists soft; exhale, and lower arms to your sides, returning to the Seated Angle Pose.**

Working your stomach muscles in the Boat Pose (Navasana)

JARGON ALERT

The Sanskrit word *Nava* means boat or ship; in this pose, you resemble a boat floating in the water. The Boat Pose is a good alternative for a full-power *vinyasa,* and it strengthens many of the muscles necessary for a progressive Power Yoga practice.

Normally, you do a *vinyasa* between each pose; but here, I have you practice this pose as an alternative to a *vinyasa.* Follow these steps to work your stomach muscles with the Boat Pose:

1. **Begin in the Seated Angle Pose — hands by your sides and legs extended in front of you; bend your knees, and place your feet flat on the floor.**

2. **Rock back on your rear as you lift your feet off the floor and extend your arms to your sides parallel to the ground; balance in this position for three complete breaths.**

3. **Straighten your legs as you lift them to form a 45-degree angle with the floor, as shown in Figure 11-6.**

   This leg-lift gives your stomach and legs an even greater workout.

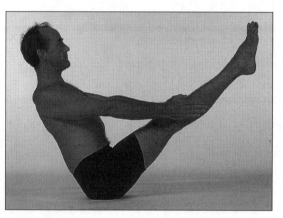

Figure 11-6: In the Boat Pose, you strengthen the muscles of your stomach, legs, and arms.

Counter-stretching with the Cobra Pose (Bhujangasana)

The Sanskrit word *Bhujanga* translates as "snake" or "serpent." In this pose, you resemble a snake slowly uncoiling as you roll back your vertebra one at a time. The Cobra Pose is an excellent counter-stretch for the Seated Forward Bend because it stretches the muscles on the front of your body.

Follow these steps to achieve the Cobra Pose:

1. **Lie on your stomach with your arms extended by your sides and your palms facing upward; turn your head to one side and then the other, and then close your eyes and relax for a few seconds.**

2. **Turn your face to the floor, and rest on your forehead; bend your elbows, and place your hands up under your shoulders.**

   Your feet should be pointed, yet relaxed.

3. **On an inhalation, slowly lift your shoulders and torso off the floor, one vertebra at a time.**

   Lift as high as is comfortable for you. If the lifting action becomes uncomfortable, rest on your elbows. If you're more flexible, lift your torso as you straighten your arms higher by extending your arms more.

   You can protect your lower back by pressing the tailbone down to engage the abdominal muscles. Keep the abs engaged as you lift your torso to prevent over-arching the lower back.

4. **When you reach your maximum comfortable stretch, remain in that position for five deep breaths.**

   Check Figure 10-3a to see what this pose looks like.

   If you have a stiff lower back, you can separate your legs a bit and allow your ankles to turn outward.

5. **Exhale, and lower your torso and shoulders to the floor; take your hands out from under your shoulders, extend your arms to your sides, turn your head to the side, and relax.**

Sitting and breathing in the Easy Posture

Before you go into a deep relaxation at the end of your Power Yoga workout, you can slow yourself down with some yogic breathing techniques. This gradual cooling off in your routine helps you to relax completely.

When you prepare for any breathing exercise, begin by finding your center and quieting your mind. You may be more comfortable and find holding a good posture easier if you sit on a small pillow rather than sitting directly on the floor or on your Yoga mat. As always, you may sit on the edge of a chair if that is more comfortable to you. The object is to be able to concentrate on your breathing, not the pain in your backside!

Follow these steps to easy breathing:

1. **Repeat the Yoga breathing exercise recommended at the beginning of this routine (refer to "Starting well is breathing well").**

2. **When you finish your Yoga breathing, lie down on your back and prepare for a wonderful journey into deep relaxation.**

Relax, why don't you?

As luxurious as deep relaxation feels, don't think of it as a "luxury" add-on to your Power Yoga practice. The deep relaxation exercise is one of the most important parts of your whole Power Yoga routine. Make sure you wrap up every Power Yoga practice with a deep relaxation exercise, or your body, mind, *and* practice will suffer. You and I both live in a fast paced society, and we can't avoid absorbing lots of stress and anxiety in our daily lives. A good, fast-paced Power Yoga workout helps to melt the effects of that tension from our muscles, but we need the relaxation phase of that workout to wash the effects of that tension from our minds. Deep relaxation is one of the simple things in life that means a lot. So don't overlook this opportunity for a mini-vacation at the end of every Power Yoga session!

Enjoying a moment of deep relaxation with the Corpse Posture (Savasana)

The Sanskrit word *Sava* (pronounced sha-va) means "corpse." In this posture, you lie flat on the floor, completely relaxed and motionless. The Corpse Posture, shown in Figure 11-7, is a great way to experience the deep relaxation phase that caps off your Power Yoga session.

In the deep relaxation phase, you release stress and tension throughout your entire body and mind. Your blood pressure decreases, your heart rate slows, and you are rewarded with a euphoric feeling that can last for hours. You also will relieve stress and tension, and create total relaxation in every fiber of your body. The deep relaxation phase promotes complete physical and mental rejuvenation as it boosts your motivation and self-esteem.

Figure 11-7:
To get the most from the Corpse Posture, pay close attention to your Yoga breathing techniques.

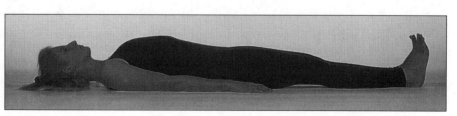

1. Lie on your back, with your arms at your sides and your legs extended.

   This is called the Corpse Pose.

2. Close your eyes, relax, and begin taking slow, deep breaths.

3. Lift your right leg about 12 inches from the floor, tense every muscle in your leg for a few seconds, relax, and then gently lower your leg to the floor; repeat this step with your left leg.

4. Tighten the muscles in your hips and buttocks for a few seconds, and then relax and let your gluteus muscles "melt" into the floor.

5. Arch your back, pressing down with your elbows and shoulders as you expand your chest toward the ceiling; hold this position for a few seconds, gently lower your back to the floor, and then relax.

6. Press your lower back into the floor by tightening your buttock and stomach muscles as you press against the floor; hold this position for a few seconds, and then relax completely.

7. Lift your right arm about 12 inches off the floor, tensing all the muscles; hold this position for a few seconds, and then relax and lower your arm to the floor; repeat this step using your left arm.

8. Roll your head slowly to the right, and then to the left; return your head to the center, and relax.

9. Fill your mouth with air, blowing your cheeks out like balloons; hold for a couple of seconds, and then relax and release the air.

10. Gently stretch all your facial muscles, and then relax them.

11. Close your eyes, take five slow, deep breaths, and clear your mind.

12. Working from your toes to your head, visualize each part of your body and tell each muscle to relax.

13. Visualize your heart, and mentally ask your heart to relax.

14. Visualize your brain, and calm it by releasing your thoughts.

15. Clear your mind of all but the most pleasant and positive thoughts.

16. After 5–30 minutes, slowly stretch your arms over your head on an inhalation and then roll over onto your right side, with your arms and legs slightly bent; remain in this position for a few breaths.

17. Gradually return to a sitting position and try to preserve the positive uplifting thoughts you created.

Congratulations! You just finished your first full-blown Power Yoga workout session. If everything went well, you should feel calm, refreshed, relaxed, and ready to go! To keep the good feelings alive, I suggest that you take a quiet walk in one of your favorite settings. Notice the world around you, and be happy that you're on the way to becoming a full-fledged Power yogi or yogini.

But don't forget the lessons from this first Power Yoga routine. For example, this session may have given you some good ideas about what kinds of props you need (or don't need) for certain kinds of postures. And you probably have a better idea of your current flexibility limits for specific postures, so you know when you might need to use some alternative moves during your Power Yoga workout (and you have some flexibility goals to work on, too).

Finally, be proud of the great job you did during this workout. I leave you with the traditional yogic blessing: Namaste. Now go enjoy yourself!

Chapter 12

Following Buddha's Way: A Moderate Power Routine

In This Chapter

▶ Getting ready for an intermediate-level workout

▶ Taking the middle road with Buddha's Way

Centuries ago, Buddha determined that the true path to enlightenment was the middle way — nothing radical or extreme, just consistent, persistent progress. I named this routine Buddha's Way, because it's an intermediate-level Power Yoga routine that offers a moderate approach to building your Power Yoga fitness.

This routine is moderate in every way; it even takes a moderate amount of time to complete. Most folks can complete this routine in about 60 minutes. The Buddha's Way routine is a bit more challenging than the Walk in the Park routine in Chapter 11, but it's a good, strong intermediate workout when you are ready to move up to the next stage of your Power Yoga practice.

Progressing along Buddha's Way

I designed the Buddha's Way routine as part of a natural progression from the simpler, less-demanding routine in Chapter 11 to the intense, high-burn workout in Chapter 13. This routine helps you build the strength and stamina that you need to keep progressing in your Power Yoga practice.

As an intermediate-level student, you may want to concentrate some of your effort on developing the "flow" of your practice. Approach the workout with confidence, and move through it at your own pace, being sure to focus on your Yoga breathing (see the Cheat Sheet or Chapter 10) throughout the routine.

These tips may help you as you move through the Buddha's Way Power Yoga workout:

✔ **Practice at your own pace:** If you find that this routine is too strenuous for you, go back to the Walk in the Park in Chapter 11 until that routine feels too easy. On the other hand, if this routine doesn't challenge you enough, feel free to progress to the advanced routine in Chapter 13. You're on your own schedule, so choose the Power Yoga practice that's best for you.

✔ **Prepare your workout environment:** Before you begin this workout session, make sure that your workout space is ready. The room should be warm and, if possible, have a good supply of fresh air. Gather your props — a yoga mat, blocks, straps, or pillows — and have them nearby.

The Intermediate Routine: Buddha's Way

This routine starts off with some Power Yoga breathing techniques, moves softly into a few warm-ups, and then provides a mild *vinyasa* (linking movement) to standing. From the standing position, you will get a taste of some powerful standing poses, and then move softly back to the floor for some traditional, finishing *asanas* (poses). Then your journey will end with breathing and deep relaxation.

Table 12-1 gives you a quick overview of the postures and *vinyasas* included in the Buddha's Way routine. The table also lists the figures that first illustrate individual postures, in case you need a refresher on the poses. After you're familiar with each exercise, you can use the table to quickly remind you of the routine's sequence.

Table 12-1	Buddha's Way Practice Routine	
Exercise	*Duration*	*Reference*
Yoga breathing	5 breaths	Cheat Sheet
Cat Chases Your Dog	2 repetitions	Figures 9-3–9-7
Downward Dog Push-Ups	5 repetitions	Figure 12-1
Missing Link Upward	1 repetition	Figures 10-13, 10-14, & 10-1c, 10-1a
Energy Saver Salutation	2–3 repetitions	Figure 10-1
Feeling Your Oats Salutation	2–3 repetitions	Figures 10-1a, 10-6–10-8
Extended Triangle	5 breaths each side	12-3
Full Warrior I	5 breaths	Figure 10-10
Warrior II	5 breaths	Figure 12-4

Exercise	Duration	Reference
Missing Link Downward	1 repetition	Figures 10-1a,10-1c,10-14b
Head to Knee	5 breaths	Figure 12-5
UFO	1 repetition	Figures 10-13, 10-11a, 10-11b, 10-12, 10-3b
Incline Plane	5 breaths	Figure 12-6
One Arm Cobra	3 repetitions	Figure 12-7
Half Vinyasa	1 repetition	Figures 10-3a, 10-3b, 10-13
Twist	5 breaths each side	Figure 12-9
Shoulder Stand	10 breaths	Figure 12-10
Fish	5 breaths	Figure 12-11
Scale	20 breaths	Figure 12-12
Yoga breathing	5 breaths	Cheat Sheet
Deep relaxation	5–10 minutes	Figure 14-1

Enough with the preliminaries — your intermediate-level Yoga routine starts here. Enjoy!

Getting off to a good start with Yoga breathing

Take a few minutes to practice your breathing before you start your Yoga exercises. This routine is a bit more demanding than the beginner-level routines, and you need to prepare your body and mind for the session ahead.

You may feel more comfortable sitting on the edge of a sturdy, non-rolling chair or on a pillow during this exercise. Either position is fine; just be certain to keep your back straight and your mind relaxed, but alert.

This exercise begins in the Easy Posture, but as you gain more experience in Power Yoga, you can substitute any of the seated positions in Chapter 8. In the course of this routine, you'll also use the Yoga breathing and the Jnana Mudra hand position from that chapter. If you need a refresher on any of these techniques, see Figure 8-4 or check the Cheat Sheet at the front of this book before you begin this routine.

Some tips for a sunnier salutation

Your goal should be to make your Sun Salutation as graceful as possible. Try to time your moves with your breathing, for the most beneficial exercise. And remember to embrace a mind-body connection as you move through the steps of the Sun Salutation. Before you move, try to visualize where your body is going, and then let your body flow in that direction. If you let your mind flow freely during the Sun Salutation, your body will follow.

Follow these steps to practice good Yoga breathing:

1. **Sit on the floor in the seated posture of your choice (see Chapter 8).**

   Try out several seated poses and work on the ones you find the most difficult.

2. **Extend your arms over your knees, resting your wrists on your knees, with your palms facing upward; form *Jnana Mudra* with your hands.**

3. **Begin your Yoga breathing; as an intermediate student, strive to lengthen the time of your inhalations and exhalations, so that you breathe more slowly and take in more oxygen.**

4. **As you breathe, visualize your lungs expanding on inhalations and contracting on exhalations.**

5. **Hold this position for 10–15 slow, deep breaths.**

   Continue your Yoga breathing throughout this session.

Letting the cat chase your dog

You begin this exercise with a little cat stretch, and then find your wild cat chasing your Downward Facing Dog up into the air. If you need a brush-up on the Downward Facing Dog Posture, check out Chapter 10, Figure 10-3b.

The Cat Chases Your Dog Stretch tones up your back muscles, strengthens your arms, and can make your entire spine feel stronger and more flexible. If you suffer from minor back pain brought on by stress, over-activity, or bad posture, this exercise can help relieve that pain and get you back in action.

Follow these steps to play cat-and-dog:

1. **Sit back on your heels, with your toes pointing back; your back should be straight, and you should feel your neck lengthen.**

2. **Lift your hips, and place your hands on the floor, so that you're resting on your hands and knees (keep your shoulders over your hands). Keep your back straight, but not rigid, gaze toward the floor, and relax as you take 3 slow, deep breaths.**

3. **On an exhalation, arch your back like a cat; relax your neck as you drop your head and gaze toward your knees (refer to Figure 9-4).**

4. **On an inhalation, lower your back and let it sway downward as you bend your arms to lower your chest and bring your chin to rest on the floor between your hands (refer to Figure 9-5).**

5. **Exhale, slowly draw your body upward, return to the arched-back position you entered in Step 3.**

6. **Straighten your arms and legs, lifting your hips to form a 90-degree angle with your body; lengthen your torso from your hands to your hips, spread your fingers, and flatten your hands firmly onto the floor.**

   This is the Downward Facing Dog Pose (see the Cheat Sheet).

7. **Roll your shoulders down toward your hips and open your chest.**

   Your feet should be about 12 inches apart, forming a solid base for this posture.

   Try to keep your feet flat on the floor, with your heels down. But if this is uncomfortable for you, don't force it; bend your knees slightly and shorten the distance between your feet and your hands.

8. **Relax your mind, and gaze toward your toes; hold this position for five slow, deep breaths.**

Warming your muscles with Downward Dog Push-Ups

Why not train your dog to do some pushups, and really turn up the heat? Downward Dog Pushups help you to build strength in your arms and shoulders. This pose helps prepare you for headstands — some of the more demanding *vinyasas* — and arm-balance exercises.

Follow these steps to warm up your dog:

1. **From the Downward Facing Dog Posture (see the Cheat Sheet), bend your elbows so that they touch the floor; rest on your forearms, and interlace your fingers.**

2. **Keep your head off the floor, and gaze toward your hands (see Figure 12-1a).**

3. **On an exhalation, lower your chin over your interlocked hands as shown in Figure 12-1b, inhale, and push yourself back to the Downward Facing Dog Posture.**

Figure 12-1:
You use the
Downward
Facing Dog
Posture to
launch
into these
push-ups.

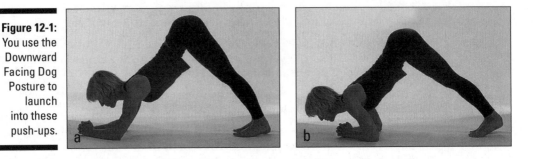

4. **Repeat Steps 1 through 3 five times, then lower your knees to the floor, bend forward at your waist, resting your torso on your thighs, with your arms stretched in front of you, palms facing downward; relax in this Child's Pose for 1–2 breaths.**

5. **Sit up slowly.**

Stretching into the Extended Triangle Pose (Utthita Trikonasana)

In Sanskrit, *utthita* means "extended or expanded," and *trikona* means "triangle." In this posture, you form an extended triangle with your body.

The Extended Triangle Pose helps relieve backaches, tones your spine, and strengthens your back. This pose also helps to strengthen your hamstrings, thigh muscles, and calf muscles.

Follow these steps to achieve the Extended Triangle Pose:

1. **Begin in the Mountain Pose I, shown in Figure 12-2; exhale completely, and on an inhalation, step your right foot out about 3½–4 feet from your left foot; at the same time, extend your arms out at your sides and parallel to the floor.**

2. **On an exhalation, pivot your right foot to the right and turn your left foot in at about a 45-degree angle; try to keep your hips and shoulders facing forward.**

3. **Still exhaling, tilt your torso to your right and lower your right hand toward the toes of your right foot.**

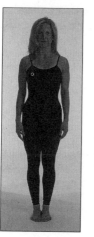

Figure 12-2:
The Mountain I posture offers a strong, well-grounded starting point for many Power Yoga exercises.

To keep your ribs extending evenly, roll your torso over the top of your thigh, creating a fold at the hip (not a rounding at the waist). It's much like folding the flap of an envelope over when sealing a letter.

4. **Grasp the big toe of your right foot with the first two fingers of your right hand.**

   If you aren't flexible enough to do this, rest your elbow on your right knee or rest your right hand on a block at the outside of your right ankle.

5. **Lift your left arm straight into the air with your palm facing outward, making a 90-degree angle with your torso; direct your gaze toward your left hand (see Figure 12-3).**

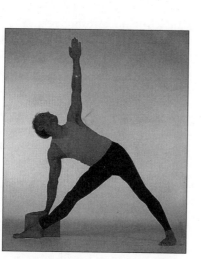

Figure 12-3:
The Extended Triangle Pose is an excellent way to keep your back in shape, expand your chest, and improve your balance, even if you use a block.

6. Continue your slow, deep Yoga breathing, and hold this position for five complete breaths; keep your torso extended over your right leg, and try to keep your chest expanded and your back flat.

7. Inhale, and lift your torso to a standing position, extending your arms out to your sides so that they are parallel to the floor.

8. Exhale, and lower your arms by your sides.

9. Repeat Steps 2 through 8 on your left side.

Stand with your feet approximately 3½–4 feet apart.

10. On an inhalation, turn both feet in to point forward; exhale, and lower your arms to your sides, and then inhale, jumping or stepping your feet back together into the Mountain Pose I.

Joining the two warriors (Virabhadrasana)

The Warrior Poses get their names from their powerful, wide stance. In Chapter 11, I use the Warrior Pose I. In this routine, I introduce Warrior Pose II to the mix. Both postures tone and strengthen your leg muscles, expand your chest, and help you develop deep, powerful breathing and good balance.

Follow these steps to achieve the Warrior Pose II:

1. Begin in the Expanded Mountain Pose, standing with your spine straight, your shoulders back, your feet about four feet apart, and your arms resting by your sides.

2. Pivot on your feet, and turn your body to the right, with your right foot facing straight to your right and your left foot at a 45-degree angle to your right foot; square your hips, shoulders, and torso to your right side, and plant your feet firmly on the ground.

3. Lunge by bending your right knee until it forms a 90-degree angle from your hamstring to your calf muscle.

Your knee should be over your heel and your thigh parallel to the floor.

4. On an inhalation, lift your arms out to your sides and over your head, keeping your arms straight, your palms together, and your fingers pointing toward the sky.

5. Drop your head, and stretch your torso upward, keeping your back foot flat on the floor.

If this is too difficult or uncomfortable, turn the toes of your left foot down and rest on your toes.

6. Hold this position for five breaths, and then lower your arms until they're parallel to the floor.

7. Remaining in your lunge position, twist your torso to the left as you extend your right arm over your right thigh and parallel to the floor; at the same time, extend your left arm behind you, over your left leg and parallel to the floor.

8. Square off your hips, shoulders, and torso to the front, in line with your arms (see Figure 12-4).

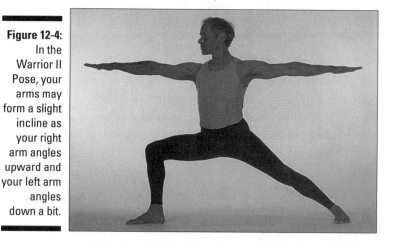

Figure 12-4: In the Warrior II Pose, your arms may form a slight incline as your right arm angles upward and your left arm angles down a bit.

9. Keep your gaze forward, along the line of your leading arm; anchor both feet firmly on the ground.

10. Hold this position for 5 complete breaths.

11. Straighten your right leg on an inhalation; drop your arms to your sides, return to the Expanded Mountain Pose (see the Cheat Sheet), and relax.

12. Repeat Steps 1 through 11 on your left side.

Moving back down with the Missing Link Downward

In this sequence, you take the Missing Link in the opposite direction, to return to the floor for your seated *asanas*. If you need a refresher on the movements for Missing Link Downward, check Chapter 10.

1. Perform the Missing Link Downward.

2. Continue your Yoga breathing.

Stretching into the Head to Knee Pose (Janu Sirsasana)

In Sanskrit, *janu* means "knee" and *sirsa* means "head." So, you won't be surprised that in this posture, you lower your head toward your knee.

The Head to Knee Pose stretches your hamstrings and calf muscles, and it helps to keep your knees flexible and strong. This exercise can also enhance the functions of your prostate gland, spleen, and kidneys.

1. **Start from the Seated Angle Pose (see the Cheat Sheet).**

2. **Keep your feet pointed upward and slightly flexed as you fold your hands in your lap.**

3. **Bend your right knee, placing your right foot against your left thigh and bringing the heel of your right foot toward your groin as you try to lower your right knee to the floor.**

   Don't push your knee past its endurance. If you can't lower your knee all the way to the ground, place a small pillow under it to provide support.

   This pose depends on flexibility in your hips, not your knees. You should feel little, if any, tugging in your knees.

4. **On an inhalation, expand your chest and lift your arms to your sides and over your head above your shoulders; let your eyes follow your hands as they rise above your head.**

   Your left leg should be extended and your foot flexed upward.

5. **Exhale, lowering your arms out and down toward your feet as you bend your torso forward and reach toward the toes of your extended left leg.**

   Keep your torso aligned with your extended left leg. If your flexibility is limited, try bending your left knee slightly and placing your hands on your left shin.

   Stay tuned into the sensations in your lower back and make sure you don't over-stretch!

6. **Take the toes of your left foot in both hands, and gently pull back on your foot.**

   If you aren't feeling that flexible, use a Yoga strap to extend your reach.

7. **Lift your elbows up; keeping them slightly bent, gaze toward your toes; hold the position for five deep breaths (see Figure 12-5).**

8. **Exhale completely; on an inhalation, return to the seated position by letting your hands slide up your leg and lifting your arms over your head.**

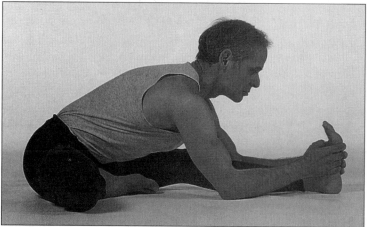

Figure 12-5:
The Head to Knee pose gives your leg muscles a great stretch and opens your hips.

9. **Exhale, and lower your arms to your sides as you straighten out your bent right leg to return to the Seated Angle Position.**

10. **Repeat Steps 1 through 9 on your other side.**

Flying on the Incline Plane (Purvottanasana)

In Sanskrit, *Purva* means "the East." In this posture, the name relates to the front side of your body (which faces East during many Hindu practices). As you might guess from its name, in this posture you stretch the muscles on the front of your body. In the United States, you often hear this called the Incline Plane.

1. **Start from the Seated Angle Position (see the Cheat Sheet).**

2. **On an inhalation, expand your chest, lifting your arms out to your sides and over your head, and keeping your wrists soft and your palms facing outward.**

3. **Exhale while lowering your arms to your sides — back to the starting position; place your hands on the floor behind your hips, and bend your knees to bring your feet toward your groin.**

4. **Inhale, and lift your hips into the air as you drop your head slightly backward and gaze toward the ceiling.**

   Your knees should be bent at a 90-degree angle and your feet flat on the floor; your arms and hands support your body, which is parallel to the floor from the knees to the shoulders. You are now in the beginner's Incline Plane (see Figure 12-6a).

5. **If this position feels challenging to you, hold it for three complete, deep breaths, and then return to the Seated Angle position.**

   To do the advanced version of this position, try to straighten your legs completely to form a straight line with your body that inclines from the floor at a 45-degree angle, like a ramp.

6. **Place your feet as close together as possible with the soles of your feet flat on the ground, and try to maintain the line of your Incline Plane; drop your head backward, and continue with your slow, deep breathing for five complete breaths (see Figure 12-6b).**

Figure 12-6: Both the beginner's Incline Plane (a) and the advanced Incline Plane (b) are excellent counter-stretches for forward bending poses.

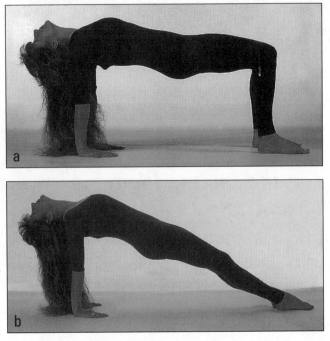

7. **Exhale, and bend at the waist to lower your hips to the floor and return to the Seated Angle Position; exhale completely, relax, and prepare to move on to the next exercise.**

Rolling into the One-Arm Cobra Pose (Bhujangasana)

The Cobra Pose helps promote good posture, expand your chest, and open stiff shoulders. The Cobra stretches all the muscles on the front of your body and builds flexibility in your spine.

1. **Lie on your stomach, with your arms along your sides and your palms facing upward; turn your head to one side, close your eyes, and relax for a few seconds.**

2. **Turn your face downward, and rest your forehead on the floor; bend your elbows, pulling them close to your body, and place your hands under your shoulders.**

   Your feet should be pointing straight behind you.

3. **On an inhalation, begin slowly lifting your shoulders and torso off the floor, one vertebra at a time, like a snake slowly uncoiling; lift as high as you comfortably can.**

   If you become uncomfortable, rest on your elbows. If you're feeling fairly flexible, lift your torso higher by extending your arms further in front of you.

   Keep your shoulders back and down, away from your ears. This is the Cobra Pose.

4. **When you reach your maximum comfortable stretch, shift your weight to your right by pivoting your right forearm inward, parallel to your shoulders and extending your left arm across your lower back.**

5. **At the same time, bend your right knee and lift your right foot toward the ceiling; try to grasp your right ankle with your left hand, as shown in Figure 12-7.**

Figure 12-7:
The One-Arm Cobra provides tension-releasing shoulder and thigh stretches.

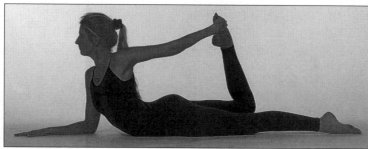

6. **Remain in this position for 5 deep breaths.**

   If you find this position too difficult, go back to Step 3 and remain in the Cobra Pose.

7. **Exhale, release your ankle, and return your torso and shoulders to the floor; as you do so, take your hands out from under your shoulders, and extend your arms back along your sides.**

8. **Turn your head to one side, and relax.**

9. **Repeat Steps 4 through 8 on the other side — reaching your right arm back behind your back and grasping your left ankle.**

Going all the way with the Half Vinyasa

You know all about those full *vinyasas,* but did you know that you also can use an abbreviated version? This half *vinyasa* is just the right size to create a little heat as you move from a facedown resting pose to a sitting position.

Follow these steps to achieve a Half *Vinyasa:*

1. **As you lie facedown, bring your hands up under your shoulders, place your palms on the floor, and move your feet up onto your toes (this is the Four Limb Staff, see Figure 10-11b).**

2. **On an inhalation, straighten your arms, lifting your torso, head and shoulders upward in a big arch toward the ceiling; push forward with your toes, and look upward.**

   This is Upward Facing Dog, check the Cheat Sheet or Figure 10-12.

3. **Exhale; keeping your arms straight, drop your head toward the floor as you lift your hips upward to move into the Downward Facing Dog, forming a ninety degree angle with your legs and torso.**

   Check the Cheat Sheet or Figure 10-3b.

4. **Bend your knees, and step or jump forward, with your arms supporting your weight; then lower your hips to the floor, and come to a sitting position with your hands on the floor beside you (see Figure 12-8).**

Figure 12-8:
This Half *Vinyasa* jumps you from the Downward Facing Dog position (a) into the Seated Angle posture (b).

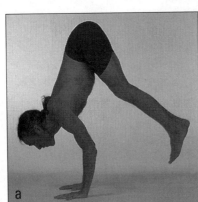

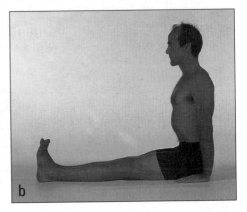

a

b

Cranking it up in the Twist Pose (Ardha Matsyendrasana)

In Hindu legend, Matsyendra was a fish that twisted around in order to hear the secrets of Yoga from Lord Siva. Matsyendra was then incarnated in human form, in order to spread the knowledge of Yoga. This posture is dedicated to Matsyendra, the twisted fish. The Sanskrit word *ardha*, meaning "half," refers to the half-twisting motion of the pose.

The Twist Pose is a great stretching and flexing exercise for your spine, and it can help relieve backaches. The Twist also stretches the muscles in your shoulders, around your ribs, and in your neck to relieve tension and leave you feeling invigorated.

Follow these steps to twist the night away:

1. **Sit on the floor with both legs extended, your spine straight, and your shoulders back.**

   This is the Seated Angle Pose (see the Cheat Sheet).

2. **Bend your right knee, and place your right foot over and beside your left leg; then, bend your left leg in to bring your left foot up toward your right hip.**

   Keep both cheeks on the floor. If this isn't possible, add a little support under the side that rises up, so that you can lengthen your back in comfort.

3. **Raise your arms, and twist your torso to the right; try to move your left elbow to the outside of your right knee.**

4. **Place your right hand on the floor behind your back for support.**

5. **Continue twisting your torso to the right and looking over your right shoulder; hold this position for five complete breaths.**

   If you're very flexible, move to Step 6; if you have limited flexibility, move to Step 7.

   Remember to lengthen, keep both shoulders down, and to enjoy the sensation.

6. **Place your left hand and arm under the bridge that you form with your right leg; reach behind your back with your left hand and try to grasp your right wrist as you continue to gaze over your right shoulder (see Figure 12-9).**

Hold this position for 5 complete breaths.

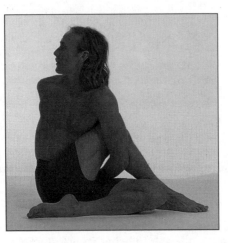

Figure 12-9:
In the Advanced Twist Pose gives your back and shoulder muscles a thorough stretch.

7. **Untwist your torso, and straighten your legs to return to the Seated Angle Position; exhale and relax.**

As you reverse the twist, release your head and neck first, then your shoulders, and finally your hips.

8. **Repeat Steps 3 through 7, this time twisting to the left (placing your left leg up and over your right leg, bending your right leg up, twisting your torso to the left, and so on).**

9. **After you return to the Seated Angle Position, relax for a few breaths, and then lie on your back.**

Moving up to the Shoulder Stand (Salamba Sarvangasana)

In Sanskrit, *salamba* means "propped or supported," *sarva* means "whole or complete," and *anga* means "limb" or "body." The English name for this posture, Shoulder Stand, may describe this pose better to a Western reader! In this posture, you support your body with your hands and elbows, and balance on your shoulders. The Shoulder Stand is what's known in the Yoga world as an *inverted pose*; inverted poses are powerful exercises that have positive effects on your entire body.

The Shoulder Stand helps to create harmony and happiness throughout your body. In this inverted *asana,* your heart and brain receive a healthy rush of blood; the pose stimulates your endocrine system and gives your thyroid and parathyroid glands a tune up. The Shoulder Stand can even help reverse the effects of varicose veins! Best of all, when you come out of the Shoulder Stand, you feel refreshed and rejuvenated.

Follow these steps to achieve the Shoulder Stand:

1. **Lie flat on your back, with your arms extended by your sides, your feet about one foot apart, your palms facing upward, and your mind calm and relaxed.**

   This is the Corpse Position.

2. **Begin your Yoga breathing, and bend your knees to pull your feet toward you, keeping them flat on the floor about one foot from your rear end.**

3. **Exhale completely, and on an inhalation, straighten your legs toward the ceiling; when your legs are straight, exhale and relax in that position.**

4. **On your next inhalation, place your hands under your hips and push down to lift your hips off the floor; tuck your elbows behind your back, and use your hands to support your elevated legs and hips.**

5. **Lift your feet toward the ceiling, tucking your chin down into your chest.**

   This is the Shoulder Stand, as shown in Figure 12-10a.

6. **Extend your legs and torso as high as you comfortably can, supporting your back with your hands.**

   Hold this posture for 5–20 slow, deep breaths.

If your neck is stiff or if you have problems getting into or maintaining this pose, lower your legs and try the pose again. This time, use a folded blanket or towel as a prop to raise your shoulders a few inches off the floor. Your head should not rest on the prop, but should hang lower than your shoulders, as shown in Figure 12-10b. The key point is that your neck doesn't support the weight of your body.

Another alternative is to start your Shoulder Stand with your legs extended up a wall and your hips resting flush against the wall; this allows you to use the wall as a prop for support (see Figure 12-10c).

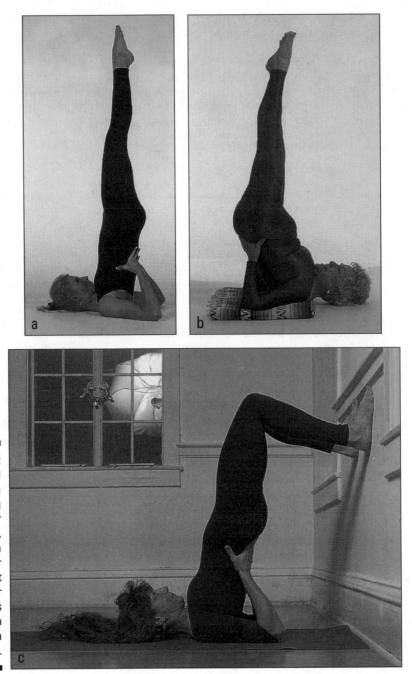

Figure 12-10:
Take a stand with a freestanding Shoulder Stand (a), one with a towel or blanket under your shoulders (b), or up against a wall (c).

Rising into the Fish Posture (Matsyasana)

In Sanskrit, *matsya* means "fish." This posture is dedicated to Matsya, the fish incarnation of *Visnu,* the "source and maintainer of all things."

The Fish Posture stretches your neck and expands your chest to help promote deep, healthy breathing. The posture also opens your hips, rejuvenates your thyroid and parathyroid glands, and helps release tension from your shoulders.

Follow these steps to achieve the Fish Posture:

1. **Lie flat on your back, with your feet about 1 foot apart and your arms extended by your sides.**

   This is the Corpse Position.

2. **Turn your palms downward, and arch your back to expand your chest.**

3. **Push down with your elbows, arms, and hands and place your hands under your hips; resting on your elbows, arch your back again to push your chest upward as you drop your head back (see Figure 12-11).**

Figure 12-11:
The object of the Fish Posture is to create a counter-stretch for the Shoulder Stand.

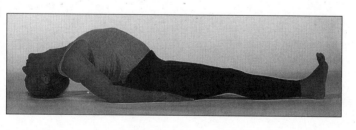

4. **Lower the top of your head to the floor.**

   If you're an advanced student, place your legs in the lotus (cross-legged) position, move your hands from beneath your hips, and rest them on the top of your thighs.

5. **Arch the front of your body as much as you can; hold this position for five slow, deep breaths.**

6. **Exhale, move your hands out from beneath you (if you didn't attempt the cross-legged position), and straighten your legs; relax into the Corpse Position for three deep breaths.**

7. **Roll onto your right side, and come to a cross-legged sitting posture.**

Weighing in on the Scale Pose (Tolasana)

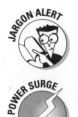

In Sanskrit, *tola* means a "pair of scales." In this *asana,* you balance your body's weight between your hands, using your shoulder muscles as the scales.

Tolasana is an excellent posture for strengthening the muscles in your stomach, arms, and shoulders. Many Power Yoga routines incorporate this posture toward the end of the session to help practitioners prepare for deep relaxation.

These steps help you balance in the Scale Pose:

1. **Sit on the floor in the Easy Posture (legs crossed) or the Lotus Posture (legs crossed and feet on opposite thighs).**

2. **Place your hands on the floor beside your hips; push down with your hands to lift your torso off the floor, as shown in Figure 12-12.**

Figure 12-12:
The Scale Pose works almost all the muscles in your body and is traditionally used toward the end of a practice session, before deep relaxation.

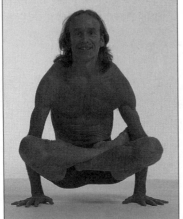

If you have difficulty lifting your body with your hands, put some Yoga blocks under your hands to give you some extra lift.

3. **While your body is suspended by your hands, lift your knees toward the ceiling and hold this position for 5–20 complete breaths.**

This movement works your stomach muscles.

4. **Lower your hips to the floor, straighten your legs, and relax.**

Congratulations! You have finished the intermediate-level Power Yoga routine with flying colors. You may want to extend the residual "good feeling" of this workout by taking a quiet walk in a favorite natural area. You'll find that the physical and mental benefits that you gained during this workout stay with you for a long time if you're aware of them (and the beauty of the world around you). In any case, I close this chapter with the traditional yogic blessing: Namaste. Have a pleasant journey!

Chapter 13

Engaging the Force:
A Full Power Routine

Some of the lead characters in the popular "Star Wars" movies acquired an internal power called the Force. Well, you don't have to be a Jedi warrior to plug into that kind of power — as a Yogi or Yogini, you can draw from your *prana,* or life-force, energy anytime (no light sabre required). And *Prana* energy is on full-tap in the routine you learn in this chapter, so get ready to embrace the vast power that lies within you!

I named this intermediate to advanced routine May the Force Be with You in honor of the powerful, vital force you nurture in your Yoga practice. This routine takes a good amount of time to complete — 60 to 90 — minutes, and it requires a lot of energy. But it also builds your strength, energy, and endurance more than any of the less advanced routines in this book — and it really burns those calories, too. So enjoy the ride, Jedi — I mean Yoga — warrior!

Moving Up to a Full-Power Routine

No question about it, May the Force Be with You is a routine for late-intermediate to advanced Yoga practitioners. At the end of this 60- to 90-minute routine, you'll understand just how hot a Power Yoga workout can be.

May the Force Be with You is a full-power routine: It generates more heat and steam than the routines in Chapters 11 and 12 (Just a Walk in the Park and Buddha's Way, respectively). This routine demands a lot, but it gives back a lot, too. In addition to the endurance and strength-building benefits of this advanced Power Yoga routine, you also benefit from its ultra-soothing relaxation.

Even after you find a routine that perfectly suits your present level of fitness, you benefit from occasionally switching back and forth between different routines (and different levels of practice).

Use these tips to get the most from this routine:

- ✔ **Set your pace:** If you find this routine too hard, go back to a less demanding routine. When you're completely comfortable with that routine, move back up to this full-level workout.

- ✔ **Step up your cross-training:** As an intermediate to advanced practitioner of Power Yoga, make sure that you continue to incorporate other kinds of physical activityinto your weekly practice. Try fast walking or running a few times a week, some long-distance or uphill bicycling, or a challenging hike. Try to move beyond the minimum of three 30-minute sessions of other physical aerobic activities every week; and don't forget to approach all of your physical activities with a yogic attitude.

- ✔ **Improve your diet and nutrition:** Consider making nutritional improvements. If you started a low-fat, high-fiber diet during your earlier Power Yoga practice, maybe it's time to look for other ways to improve your eating habits. See Chapter 22 for suggestions on how to do this.

Practicing at Full Power: May the Force Be with You

May the Force Be with You is a full-power, 60 to 90-minute routine for intermediate to advanced Power Yoga practitioners. Table 13-1 gives you a quick overview of all of the postures and *vinyasas* included and lists the chapters and figure numbers where individual postures are described in case you need to return to those original instructions for a refresher on the poses.

If you discover that this routine is too difficult for you, don't forget to move back to the Buddha's Way routine for a few weeks, and try this full-power workout again later. If you find you can't finish the routine in the estimated amount of time, just move to the cool-down exercises, then finish the rest of the routine during your next practice session.

Table 13-1	**May the Force Be with You Routine**	
Exercise	*Duration*	*Reference*
Yoga Breathing	5 breaths	"Starting Off with Yoga Breathing"

Exercise	Duration	Reference
Missing Link Upward *Vinyasa*	1 repetition	Figures 10-13, 10-14, 10-1c
Feeling Your Oats Salutation	5 repetitions	Figures 10-1a, 10-6–10-8
Mother Lode Salutation	5 repetitions	Figures 10-1a, 10-9, 10-1c, 10-7, 10-8, 10-12, 10-3, 10-10
Extended Triangle	5 breaths each side	Figure 12-3
Twisted Extended Triangle	5 breaths each side	Figure 13-1
Extended Side Angle	5 breaths each side	Figure 13-2
Flying Warrior	5 breaths each leg	Figure 13-3
Downward *Vinyasa*	1 repetition	Figures 13-4a, 13-4b, 13-5, 10-12, 10-3b, 8-1
Seated Angle	5 breathes	Cheat Sheet
Half *Vinyasa* (p. 182)	1 repetition	Figures 10-11b, 10-12, 10-3b, 12-8ab
Half Locust and Full Locust	5 breaths each	Figure 13-7
Half *Vinyasa* (p. 206)	1 repetition	Figures 10-12, 10-3b, 10-13
Wheel	5 breaths/2 repetitions	Figure 13-8
Handstand	5 breaths/2 repetitions	Figure 13-9
Shoulder Stand	10–20 breaths	Figure 12-10
Bridge	5 breaths	Figure 13-10
Headstand	10–20 breaths	Figure 13-11
Scale	30 breaths	Figure 12-12
Power Breathing	5 breaths	This chapter
Deep Relaxation	5–20 minutes	Figure 14-1

Before you begin this routine, don't forget to prepare your workout area: if you're indoors, make sure your room is warm and well-ventilated. Indoors or outdoors, be sure to have your props (Yoga mat, straps, blocks, pillows, and so on) nearby. With your tools in order, you're ready to begin your workout!

Starting Off with Yoga Breathing

As an advanced student, you need to take a few extra minutes to practice your breathing before you start your Power Yoga exercises. Expand the length of your inhalations and exhalations to create softness and power with each confident breath. Focus your thoughts as you practice your breathing techniques, and let your breathing become a meditation.

1. **Sit on the floor in the Easy Posture or any of the other seated postures in Chapter 8.**

   As you move from an intermediate to an advanced level of practice, try to use the poses you find most difficult.

2. **Extend your arms over your knees and rest your wrists on your knees, with palms facing upward. Form *Jnana Mudra* with your hands (see the Cheat Sheet or Chapter 8).**

3. **Take slow, deep breaths.**

   Visualize a beautiful, natural setting to help you reach a controlled, relaxed rhythm in your breathing.

   Remember to maintain *ujjayi* (victorious) breathing throughout your routine (check out Chapter 7 for a refresher.) As you breathe in through your nose, the in-coming air makes a soft, hissing sound on the back of your throat; as you exhale through your nose, you hear the sound of your breath vibrating against the back of your throat.

4. **Choose a *vinyasa* to transport you to standing. Continue your Yoga breathing as you move on to the next exercise.**

The victory of victorious breathing

Chapter 7 explains the techniques for *ujjayi* Yoga breathing. As an intermediate-to-advanced student, you can expect to gain even more power from practicing this breathing technique. Not only does *ujjayi* breathing help you take more oxygen into your lungs to help you move through high-throttle advanced Power Yoga exercises, but the technique also leaves you feeling more refreshed, invigorated, and powerful. The tranquil, meditative sound of Yoga breathing, in combination with your slow, deep, measured inhalations and exhalations contribute to the calming of your body and mind. Yoga breathing helps you to center your thoughts on your practice and ignore all other distractions. All things considered, victorious breathing is a winner!

Taking the UFO Vinyasa to a Standing Position

To get from your seated breathing position, you need a *vinyasa* to transport you to a standing position. As an intermediate to advanced student, I suggest the hot UFO *Vinyasa* in Chapter 10. Because you need to add a few variations to that *vinyasa* to reach a standing pose, I'll quickly run through the steps below; if you need more of a refresher on this or any other *vinyasa*, you can take a quick look at Chapter 10.

1. **Start from the Seated Angle pose, and engage your *Mula Bandha* and *Uddiyana Bandha* (see the Cheat Sheet for all three).**

   Let the sound of your Yoga breathing help you focus your attention on your movements during this jump back *vinyasa*.

2. **Bend your knees about chest high with your ankles crossed, inhale as you lift your hips up off the floor, and pivot your whole torso. Lower your chest and head toward the floor in front of you as you extend your legs behind you.**

3. **Glide your legs back into a smooth landing, with legs and arms fully extended in the Plank position.**

   Your arms should be fully extended, as if you just did a pushup; your body should be rigid like a plank.

4. **Bend your arms and lower your torso down into the Four Limb Staff position: elbows bent, chest touching the floor, supporting yourself with your hands and the toes of your flexed feet. (See Figure 10-8.)**

   If you need a boost during your jump back *vinyasa* from Seated Angle to Plank Pose, use a pair of Yoga blocks as props under your hands. You can use the same blocks to aid you in the *vinyasa* when you jump back through to Seated Angle Pose.

5. **Lift your torso on an inhalation into the Upward Facing Dog posture, with your torso arched, your chest expanded, and your gaze directed toward the sky.**

   (See the Cheat Sheet for both Upward Facing Dog and the Downward Facing Dog in Step 6.)

6. **Drop your head down and lift your hips into the air on an exhalation, into Downward Facing Dog.**

7. **Lift your torso up and jump your feet in for a safe landing between your hands.**

8. **Exhale when you land your feet, and move into the Standing Forward Bend (see the Cheat Sheet).**

9. **Inhale and expand your chest as you start to come to a standing position. Lift your arms out to your sides and up over your head. When you reach a full standing position, exhale and lower your arms down by your sides into Mountain Pose I, and then relax.**

Sun Salutation for Levels II and III

As you finish your hot UFO *Vinyasa*, you're ready to move into some powerful Sun Salutations. Do five repetitions each of the "Spicy" versions of the Level II, Feeling Your Oats, and Level III, Mother Lode Sun Salutations. I describe both of these salutations in detail in Chapter 10.

To get the most benefit from your practice, remember these Sun Salutation tips:

✔ **Time your movements with your breathing.** As an advanced student, your Sun Salutation takes on a powerful, yet graceful flow. You can enhance this process by timing your moves with your breathing.

✔ **Maintain a strong mind-body connection.** Visualize where you're going before you move to condition your body to flow from one position to the next. Become one with your movements and try to feel a connection with the power of the earth. Your Sun Salutations will generate enormous amounts of vital life force energy; try to be aware of and draw upon this energy.

Even though you are progressing into the advanced levels of Power Yoga practice, don't push your body beyond its limits. If you find it too difficult to practice 5 repetitions of Level II Salutation and Five repetitions of Level III Salutation, cut back to 3 of each until you build up endurance.

After you have completed your Sun Salutations, remain standing and follow the next set of instructions.

Stretching with the Extended Triangle and Twisted Extended Triangle Poses

The Extended Triangle Pose is a wonderful stretching exercise. In that pose, you form a triangle with your body by stretching off to the side with your torso, legs, and arms.

This basic triangle pose gives you a great stretch along the sides of your torso and opens your chest. As a bonus, the Extended Triangle strengthens your legs and helps improve your balance. What more could you want from one posture?

Well, you *can* get more from the basic triangle pose by following it up with its twisted sister, the Twisted Extended Triangle, or *Parivrtta Trikona*. In the Sanskrit language, *parivrtta* means "twisted or revolved" and *trikona* means "triangle." As you may have guessed from its name, in this posture you twist your torso as you form an extended triangle.

The Twisted Extended Triangle helps relieve backaches, tones your spine, and strengthens your back. It's also a good exercise for strengthening your hamstring, thigh, and calf muscles.

1. **Follow the steps for Extended Triangle in Chapter 12, doing 5 breaths on each side.**

2. **Go into Expanded Mountain Posture (see the Cheat Sheet).**

3. **On an exhalation, twist your torso to the left, point your left foot out at a 90-degree angle and pivot your right foot in at 45-degree angle.**

4. **Inhale, lifting your arms up and twisting your whole torso down and to the left, then exhale as you lower your right hand down and place it on the floor to the outside of your left foot.**

   If you're not quite flexible enough to reach the floor with your right hand, rest your right elbow on your left knee. Alternatively, you can rest your hand on a Yoga block placed to the right of your left foot.

   Try to keep your hips squared with the direction your left foot is pointing (don't let one hip lead the other) and keep your lower back flat.

5. **As you twist your torso, lift your left arm up perpendicular to the floor, with your palm open and facing away from your body. Gaze toward your left hand and hold this position for five slow, deep breaths (see Figure 13-1).**

Figure 13-1:
The twisting motion of the Twisted Extended Triangle builds upon the stretching and strengthening benefits of the Extended Triangle.

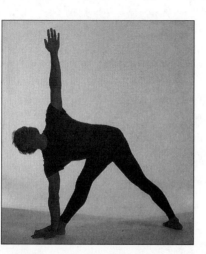

6. **Exhale all your air, then, on an inhalation come back to a standing position, lifting your torso and arms up, as you return to the Expanded Mountain Pose.**

7. **Repeat Steps 2 through 5 on your right side.**

Stretching Even Farther in the Extended Side Angle Pose (Uttihita Parsvakonasana)

In the Sanskrit language, *utthita* means "stretched or extended," *parsva* means "side or flank," and *kona* relates to the term "angle." In this pose, you form an extended side angle.

1. **Start from the Extended Mountain Pose (see the Cheat Sheet).**

2. **Turn your right foot outward ninety degrees and turn your left foot in at a forty-five degree angle. Inhale, lifting your arms up at your sides and parallel to the floor.**

3. **Exhale as you lunge down, bending your right knee.**

   Your right leg forms a ninety degree angle with your knee over your heel and your thigh parallel to the floor.

4. **Place your right hand on the floor to the right of your right foot.**

   Don't try to force yourself into this posture; just as I recommended in the Twisted Extended Triangle pose, use a prop or rest your elbow on your knee if you aren't flexible enough to reach the floor with your hand.

5. **Form a forty-five degree angle with your body: from your left extended leg (which is behind you) through your torso and all the way out to the fingertips of your left hand.**

   Your left arm is extended up at a forty-five degree angle on the same plane as your left leg and torso; your palm should be open, and your hand facing downward.

6. **Turn your head up, looking under your left arm toward the ceiling; hold this position for five slow deep breaths (see Figure 13-2).**

7. **Lift your left arm perpendicular to the floor, as you push up off the floor with your right leg. Straighten your right leg to return to the Expanded Mountain pose, with your arms out parallel to the floor. Exhale and lower your arms to your sides.**

8. **Repeat Steps 2 through 7 on your left side.**

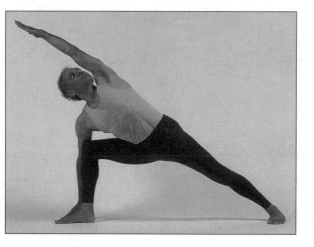

Figure 13-2:
The Extended Side Angle Pose strengthens your legs while it tones your ankles, knees, and thighs.

Moving on to Warrior III (Virabhadrasana)

This *asana* (pose) is named after Virabhdra, a powerful hero in Hindu legend. In this posture, you stand strong and powerful on one leg. As with Warrior I and II, this variation is a wonderful way to strengthen and tone the leg muscles and enhance your balance.

1. **Start from the Expanded Mountain Pose (see the Cheat Sheet).**

2. **Pivot on your feet and turn your whole body to the right side, your right foot facing straight to your right and your left foot angled in toward your right foot at a 45-degree angle. Square your hips, shoulders and torso off to your right side and plant your feet firmly on the ground.**

3. **Bend your right knee and lunge down onto your right leg with your knee forming a 90-degree angle.**

   Your knee should be over your heel and your thigh parallel to the floor.

4. **On an inhalation lift your arms out to your sides and up over your head. Straighten your arms, touch your palms together, and point toward the sky.**

5. **Lean forward and balance all your weight on your right leg.**

   Your whole body should be balancing parallel to the floor, supported only by your right foot. Your arms are extended in front of you, with your palms together and your vision directed down toward the floor as shown in Figure 13-3.

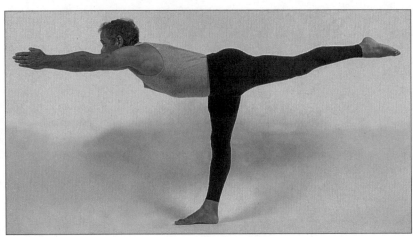

Figure 13-3:
You look as if you're flying in the Flying Warrior Pose.

6. **Hold this position for 5 slow deep breaths.**

   This is a difficult posture, and if you're very uncomfortable with it try positioning yourself in front of a wall and placing your hands flat against the wall for support. This modification works quite well.

7. **Hold this position for 5 complete breaths.**

8. **On an inhalation, bend your right knee and slowly lower your left leg back to the floor. Raise your torso and return to the Expanded Mountain Pose.**

9. **Repeat Steps 2 through 8 on your left side.**

Full UFO Vinyasa Downward (Hot Vinyasa)

In this linking movement you take the Full UFO *Vinyasa* in the opposite direction, to return you to the floor for your seated *asanas.* This is called a Full UFO *vinyasa* because it transports you from a standing to a sitting position.

The Full UFO *Vinyasa* is a hot *vinyasa,* and as such it takes a lot of energy and generates great heat and energy. This *vinyasa* comes in handy on many occasions throughout your Power Yoga practice, as it helps you keep the flow of energy moving in your routines.

1. **From Mountain Pose I (see the Cheat Sheet), lift your arms out to the sides of your body as you inhale and expand your chest. Continue lifting your arms all the way up over your head, then touch your palms together and gaze up at your hands.**

   You're in Mountain III Pose as shown in Figure 13-4a).

2. **Bend forward on an exhalation, keeping your chest open, and lower your arms out to the side then down to the floor beside your feet into a Standing Forward Bend (See figure 13-4b).**

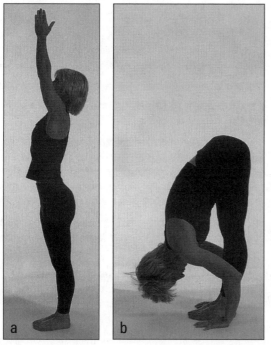

Figure 13-4:
Be sure to direct your gaze toward your hands in Mountain III (a) as you move into the full Standing Forward Bend (b).

a   b

3. **Bend your knees and jump both legs back to land in a push-up position called the Plank (see Figure 13-5).**

   Keep your body firm and solid, like a plank or board.

   If this position is too hard for you, try resting your knees on the floor. As you become more practiced in this posture, move into the full Plank position.

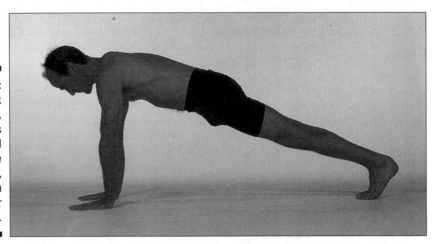

Figure 13-5:
In the Plank position, your body is rigid and strong, like a strong, wooden plank or board.

4. **Exhale and lower your body to the floor, moving into the Four Limb Staff Position (see the Cheat Sheet).**

5. **Pull your torso forward with your arms, as you inhale and push up with your feet. Arch your body upward, moving into the Upward Facing Dog Pose (see the Cheat Sheet). Push forward, rolling up onto the tops of your feet, lifting your torso upward, expanding your chest, and opening your shoulders. Direct your gaze up toward the sky.**

6. **On an exhalation, lift your hips into the air as you drop your head and shoulders down, moving into the Downward Facing Dog Pose (see the Cheat Sheet).**

7. **Spread your fingers out wide, roll your shoulders outward. Your arms and legs should be fully extended, your chest open, and your gaze directed toward your toes. Keep your feet about 1 foot apart and your heels on the floor.**

If you have trouble with this stretch, walk your feet closer to your hands and bend your knees slightly.

8. **Look up between your hands, bend your knees, and step or jump your legs and your whole torso forward (see Figure 13-6) so that you land in a Seated Angle Pose (see the Cheat Sheet).**

If jumping through your hands into a seated posture seems impossible, try using blocks under your hands to get more clearance *and* to build your arm strength. You can just step your feet up between your hands, then sit down on the floor and extend your legs in front of you.

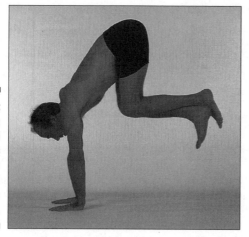

Figure 13-6:
Jumping through to sitting takes arm strength and muscle control.

Settling into Seated Angle II (Upavistha Konasana)

In the Sanskrit language, the word *upavishta* means "seated" and *kona* means "angle." In this posture, you form a seated angle with your body, but you incorporate more movement and stretching than is involved in the basic Seated Angle posture. This posture opens your hips and gives a great stretch to your hamstring and calf muscles.

1. **Sit on the floor in the Seated Angle Pose (see the Cheat Sheet).**

2. **Separate your legs as far as possible without causing strain or muscle pull.**

   You want to feel as if you are getting a stretch, but don't go so far as to cause injury.

3. **Place your hands on your thighs, and sit up with your spine straight and your shoulders back.**

4. **On an inhalation, lift your arms up over your head and touch your palms.**

5. **Exhale and bend as far forward as you need to in order to achieve a good stretch.**

6. **Hold this position for 5 complete breaths.**

7. **Inhale and lift your torso back to a sitting position.**

   As you sit up, lift your arms up over your head and touch your palms.

8. **Exhale, lower your arms back down to your sides, and move your legs back together in the Seated Angle position.**

Linking with a Modified UFO or Rolling Stone Vinyasa

You need to create little more steam now, so take another *vinyasa* here. From your Seated Angle pose, move into either the UFO or Rolling Stone *vinyasa;* you can find steps for both *vinyasas* in Chapter 10.

Work through the steps for either *vinyasa* using these variations:

- ✔ For the Rolling Stone *vinyasa,* follow Steps 1 through 5 to end up in the Downward Facing Dog position. Then, lower your torso to the floor, extend your arms down by your side with palms up, turn your head to the side and relax.

- ✔ For the UFO *vinyasa,* follow Steps 1 through 4 to end up in the Downward Facing Dog position. Then, lower your torso to the floor, extend your arms down by your side with palms up, turn your head to the side and relax.

Extending into the Half Locust (Ardha Salabhasana) or Full Locust Pose

In the Sanskrit language, *ardha* means "half" and *Salabha* is the word for "locust." In this posture you feel the energy of the earth as you rest on your stomach like a locust resting in the grass.

This posture really helps to strengthen the lower back and can be very valuable in relieving back pain, as it also enhances proper alignment of your spinal disc. The Locust Pose helps relieve flatulence, and the Full Locust has the added benefit of relieving tension in your neck muscles.

Follow these steps to work through the Half Locust.

1. **Lie on your stomach with your arms by your sides. Rest your chin on the ground as though you are trying to look out in front of you.**

2. **Place your hands (palms facing downward) underneath your thighs.**

3. Exhale all your air and then on an inhalation, lift your right leg backward and upward, pressing your left foot into the floor (see Figure 13-7a).

4. Hold this position for 5 very slow deep breaths.

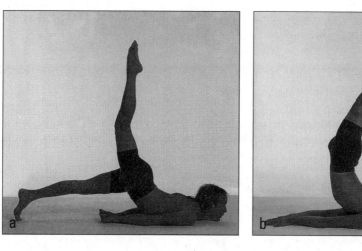

Figure 13-7:
The Half Locust posture (a) and the Full Locust (b) relieve lower back pain and strengthen the back.

5. Exhale and lower your right leg back down to the floor and relax.

6. Repeat Steps 1 through 5 lifting your left leg back and up.

7. Take your hands out from underneath your body and rest your arms by your sides. Turn your head to the side and relax for a few breaths.

If you're really strong and flexible, you may want to give the Full Locust posture a try. This posture really demands that you have a great deal of back flexibility and abdominal strength.

1. Follow Steps 1 and 2 for the preceding Half Locust position.

2. On an inhalation bend your knees, lifting both feet and legs at the same time. Push down into the floor with your arms as you lift your whole torso vertical to the floor (See Figure 13-7b).

3. Hold this position for 5 slow deep breaths.

4. Come down slowly, take your hands out from underneath you, turn your head to the side, and relax on your stomach.

Building heat with a Half Vinyasa

Up to this point in this routine, you've worked with full *vinyasas* to build heat. Here, you use a half *vinyasa,* which works nicely to create a little movement and heat as you move from a stomach-resting posture to a seated pose.

1. **From lying on your stomach at the end of your Full or Half Locust position, move your hands up under your shoulders and raise your feet up onto your toes.**

2. **On an inhalation, straighten your arms, lifting your torso, head and shoulders upward, toward the ceiling, pushing forward with your toes into Upward Facing Dog (see the Cheat Sheet).**

3. **Exhale and drop your head down toward the floor as you lift your hips upward, moving into the Downward Facing Dog (see the Cheat Sheet).**

4. **Step or jump your legs up between your hands, landing in the Seated Angle Pose (see the Cheat Sheet).**

Bending into the Wheel Pose or Upside Down Bow (Urdhva Dhanurasana)

The word *urdhva* means "upward" and *dhanu* means "bow." In this posture, you form an upside-down bow. In America, this posture is often called the Wheel Posture — sometimes it's also referred to as a plain old Backbend.

The Upside Down Bow or Wheel posture is excellent for creating a supple spine, expanding your chest, and strengthening your arms. This inverted pose also sends your brain a fresh supply of oxygenated blood, leaving you feeling very relaxed and refreshed.

1. **From the Seated Angle pose (see the Cheat Sheet), lie back on the ground and extend your arms by your sides, palms up; your feet should be about 12 inches apart (this is the Corpse Pose, also on the Cheat Sheet).**

2. **Bend your knees and draw your feet up toward your hips, keeping your feet flat on the ground.**

3. **Raise your hands up by your ears and tuck your hands, palms down, under your shoulders.**

4. **Exhale all of your air, and then inhale and push down with your hands, trying to roll back up on top of your head. (Be careful in this step, which is hard if you have a weak neck.) Simultaneously, lift your hips up into the air and arch your back, as shown in Figure 13-8a.**

5. **Continue pushing up with your hands and feet. Straighten your elbows and raise your hips until your body forms a large arc or wheel, as shown in Figure 13-8b.**

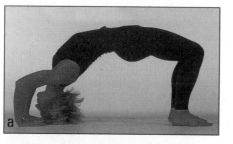

Figure 13-8:
You strengthen your arms, shoulders, and wrists practicing either the preliminary version of the Wheel Posture (a) or the more advanced version (b).

6. **Hold this position for 5–10 slow, deep breaths.**

7. **Exhale and bend your elbows to lower your head down and then softly relax your whole body back down into the Corpse position.**

ALTERNATIVE

This wheel keeps on turning

You can do a number of variations of the Wheel position — in fact, everyone can find some version of this pose that works for him or her. For example, the Bridge Posture later in this chapter is a beginner's version of the Wheel. But even if you choose the intermediate or advanced Wheel Postures, you can call on some Yoga tricks to help you swing into this backbend.

For example, you can place two wooden blocks up against a wall, turn around backwards, and lay down on the ground with your head facing the wall, place your hands on top of the blocks, then lift up into the Wheel Pose. Elevating your hands makes this pose quite a bit easier. Hold this for 5 complete deep breaths, then lower yourself back down to the ground. So, now you know that there's more than one way to bend your back!

Pushing up into a Handstand (Adho Mukha Vrksasana)

In the Sanskrit language the words *adho mukha* mean "facing downwards" and *vrksa* means "tree." In this posture, you resemble an upside-down tree with its roots up in the air. In America, this pose is called the Handstand (a name that, while less evocative than Downward Facing Tree, makes a lot more sense to us English-speaking types).

The handstand builds strength and balance as it develops your chest and strengthens your shoulders, arms, and wrist. And, as you may remember from your childhood, it's a lot of fun, too!

Fun element aside, if you haven't done a handstand before, you probably should have a friend to assist you in getting (and staying) vertical in your first attempt. If you lose your balance and crash to the ground too often, you'll soon grow tired and discouraged.

By following these steps, you'll come to a full handstand, with your feet resting up against a wall for support.

1. **Start from the Downward Facing Dog position (see the Cheat Sheet), with your hands located a few inches away from a wall and your fingers spread wide.**

2. **Bend your left knee and step your left leg forward about 2 feet behind your hands.**

3. **Use your bent left leg to jump your body up off the floor, throwing your weight onto your arms and hands. Keep your arms straight, drop your head down, and lift your hips upward. Straighten your legs up into the air and rest your feet against the wall, as shown in Figure 13-9a.**

4. **Hold this posture for 5 deep breaths.**

   If you're confident of your balance, you can work on holding your handstand without the support of a wall as Figure 13-9b shows.

5. **Repeat twice for a total of three repetitions.**

6. **Bring your feet back to earth and lie on your back.**

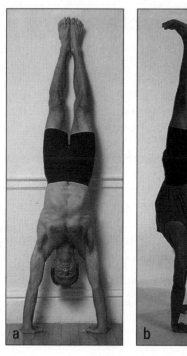

Figure 13-9:
Use the wall
or a friend
to help you
do a
Handstand
(a), or do a
freestanding
one (b).

More Inversions with the Shoulder Stand (Salamba Sarvangasana)

The Shoulder Stand stimulates your endocrine system and gives your thyroid and parathyroid glands a tune-up. As with the Handstand, this posture floods your brain with fresh oxygenated blood and helps reverse the effects of varicose veins. When you come out of the Shoulder Stand, you feel refreshed and rejuvenated. This ready supply of oxygenated blood and the powerful feeling it conveys make this posture an important part of any advanced Power Yoga routine.

Chapter 12 provides step-by-step directions for assuming the Shoulder Stand pose. Follow the instructions there, referring to Figure 12-10, then prepare for the counter-stretching motion of the Bridge Posture — the next pose.

Building the Bridge Posture (Setu Bandhasana)

Setu means "bridge," and *setu bandha* means the "construction of a bridge." In this posture, you form the shape of a bridge with your torso, using your arms as supports. This is an excellent stretch for the muscles of the chest, arms, and thighs. You also feel a release of tension in your lower back.

1. **Lie in the Corpse position (see the Cheat Sheet).**

2. **Bend your knees up, and place your feet flat on the floor. Raise your hips off the floor and stretch your arms under your back, with your palms facing down. (Advanced students, grab your ankles with your hands.)**

3. **Leave your head, shoulders, and feet on the floor, and push your torso up with your thighs (see Figure 13-10).**

   You should resemble a bridge over a river.

4. **Hold this position for 5–10 slow, deep breaths.**

Figure 13-10:
The Bridge Posture stretches your thighs and pelvis and encourages really deep Yoga breathing.

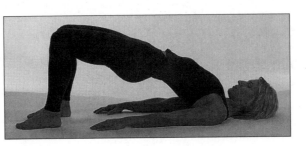

5. **Take your hands out from underneath you and lower your hips to the floor, and return to Corpse posture.**

Reversing course with the Headstand (Salamba Sirsasana)

In Sanskrit, the word *salamba* means "supported" and *sirsa* means "head." In this inverted posture, you support your headstand with your elbows and forearms.

The big benefits of inverted postures

The Headstand, Shoulder Stand, Handstand, and other upside-down Yoga postures are more than just your average cool-looking *asanas*. These inverted postures bring some unique benefits to your Power Yoga routine. Of course, they help you develop balance, and they're also great for building your strength — and confidence. But by their very nature, inverted postures also work wonders on your body's cardiovascular system. We all spend many hours each day with our bodies in an upright position. When you turn your body upside down, you ease the flow of blood to your heart and brain. Combined with your deep Yoga breathing (which ups the oxygen supply to your blood),

this flush of fresh, oxygenated blood coursing through your heart and brain leaves you feeling refreshed and powerful. And inverted Yoga postures can also help prevent and ease the symptoms of varicose veins. All things considered, you should be sure to include a few inverted postures in every Power Yoga routine — it's good to look at your workout from a new perspective, right?

Warning: Check with your doctor before practicing inverted postures if you have high blood pressure, serious eye injury, and/or you're menstruating.

1. **From the Corpse Posture, roll over on your stomach, bring your hands under your shoulders, and push up to raise your body to rest on your hands and knees.**

2. **Bend your elbows, lower your body onto your forearms, and interlace your fingers (leaving your hands cupped).**

3. **Lower your head until you can place your cupped hands around the back of your head as shown in Figure 13-11a).**

4. **Supporting most of your weight on your elbows, straighten your legs very slowly, distributing half your weight on your head and elbows and half on your feet.**

5. **Slowly walk your feet up toward your face a little bit higher and hold this position doing your slow deep breathing. (See Figure 13-11b.)**

Figure 13-11: These preliminary steps help you move slowly and smoothly into a full headstand.

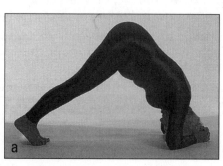
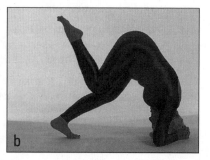

If you're not ready yet for the full headstand, follow Steps 6 through 8. To power on to the full headstand, move to Step 9.

6. **Walk your feet away from your face about six inches.**

7. **Shift your weight off your torso back toward your feet, lifting your head off the floor, as you put all your weight on your elbows. Move your head back in the direction of your elbows.**

   You're now resting on your forearms, elbows, and feet with your fingers interlaced and your head dangling.

8. **After a couple of breaths with your head hanging and your body forming a ninety degree angle to the floor, exhale and shift your hips forward as you lower your head slowly down between your hands. Go to step 13.**

9. **To go into the full Headstand, from the position in Step 4, walk your feet up higher until your torso is almost vertical.**

10. **Bend your right knee and tuck it into your chest, taking your foot up off the floor (see Figure 13-11b), then bend your left knee into your chest as you pull your left foot up off the floor.**

If you aren't completely confident about your balance, try the headstand with your back against a wall for added support. In Step 1, position your head 5 or 6 inches away from the wall, and at Step 9 kick one leg up and place that foot on the wall. Then, kick your other leg up and use both feet (keeping your knees slightly bent) to help balance you in your headstand.

11. **Lift your legs up into a full Headstand, as shown in Figure 13-12.**

   Whether you're using a wall for support or your Headstand is freestanding, support most of the weight on your elbows and forearms and very little on your head.

12. **Tuck your hips under, flatten your back, and try to form one straight line from your head through your shoulders, spine, legs, and toes. Avoid arching your back and pushing your belly out, or you could put strain on your back muscles.**

13. **Hold your headstand for at least 10 slow, deep breaths. But don't force yourself to hold the position if it becomes uncomfortable.**

14. **After your breathing, or when the position becomes uncomfortable, come down slowly by bending your knees into your chest and lowering your torso back down onto your thighs.**

15. **Extend your arms out in front of you in Child's Pose (see the Cheat Sheet), and relax in this position for 10 breaths.**

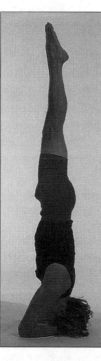

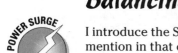

Figure 13-12:
Try a full
Headstand
only if
you're very
confident of
your
balance.

Balancing with the Scale Pose (Tolasana)

I introduce the Scale pose in the Buddha's Way routine in Chapter 12. As I mention in that chapter, the Scale pose is a "frequent flyer" in Power Yoga — it's used toward the end of many routines and followed by deep relaxation.

Go through the steps and refer to Figure 12-12 to do the Scale pose.

Sitting and breathing in Easy Posture

Before you go into the deep relaxation exercise that caps this routine, take this moment to slow yourself down with some more Yoga breathing techniques. A gradual slow-down helps you relax totally and completely when you move on to the deep relaxation.

Find your center and quiet your mind; then, follow Steps 1 through 4 of the Yoga breathing exercise you used to begin this routine (see "Starting off with Yoga Breathing").

Capping Your Routine with Deep Relaxation (Savasana)

Deep Relaxation is one of the most important exercises in your whole Power Yoga routine. Especially after this high-powered workout, your body and mind need the refreshing and calming touch of total relaxation. Don't let this exercise's simplicity fool you into thinking it isn't worthwhile. You need it — and you'll like it!

I give you the detailed steps for the Deep Relaxation exercise in Chapter 14. Follow those steps — and remember to take at least 5 minutes for this exercise (more, if possible).

Well, how does it feel to realize that you've now completed a full-power, advanced Power Yoga routine? You should feel great — alive, energetic, flexible, and (most of all) confident and at peace. *Remember:* Vary your routine levels, by occasionally returning to less advanced workouts, such as those I describe in Chapters 11 and 12. But always take some time to enjoy your Power Yoga accomplishments as you look back over how much you've advanced in your practice!

Now, relax, take a nice, quiet walk, and keep the good feelings alive. Namaste, have a pleasant journey!

Chapter 14

Dialing Down the Power

- -

In This Chapter

▶ Embracing the benefits of deep relaxation

▶ Merging power with stillness

▶ Touching your soul with meditation

- -

In order to replenish your full power, you need to rest and conserve your energy from time to time. I know, I know — you live in a fast-paced world, where time is money and a need for rest is considered a sign of weakness. Get over it. As a Power Yoga student, you discover the importance of feeding your body with good air, good food, good exercise, and good rest.

In this chapter, you discover ways to restore your body. I show you the proper way to relax (did you know that there is an art to taking it easy?), then I take you one step further and demonstrate ways to enhance your rest by controlling your "rest-less" mind through meditation. I explore different types of meditation, and the best way to combine meditation with your Power Yoga practice. As you restore your waking mind and body, you actually improve the quality of the rest you get when you're asleep. So stretch your arms and settle back for a lively look at rest.

Cooling Down

It's most important that you take the time to relax and cool down after your Power Yoga workout. Capping your practice with relaxation gives your body *and* mind a chance to cool down and absorb the energy and power you generate during your workout. A proper cooling-down leaves you feeling refreshed and invigorated by your workout — not exhausted.

If you're used to living life in the fast lane, you may have to force yourself to take time for relaxation exercises at the end of your workout. If that's the case, you probably need that relaxation time more than you know. If you want to operate at full power, you need to recharge your batteries. So just do it!

Cooling down gradually is best; reduce the intensity and speed of your exercises as you get toward the end of your session (and don't forget to practice your Yoga breathing exercises). Use the deep relaxation technique I show you in this chapter to end your session. As you tense and relax each muscle, you find your body and mind drawn deeper into a complete state of relaxation. At the end of your deep relaxation phase you'll be refreshed and ready to tackle the rest of your busy day.

Relaxing for the Health of It

Relaxation releases stress, tension, and fatigue from every part of your body. And, it eases and quiets your mind, leaving you feeling calm yet alert and ready to respond to the world around you. Giving your body and mind proper relaxation is the best way to buffer your stress threshold, so that you react more calmly to the never-ending ups and downs of daily life.

Yes, Power Yoga helps you *avoid* stress. You first notice this when you fall out of a balanced pose and smile. Yes, smile! You don't even miss a breath, you just calmly regain your balance and move on through your practice, the picture of tranquility. You notice it next when something happens that usually drives you nuts — say, losing your keys. If your normal response is ranting and raving as you tear around the house feverishly searching, get ready for a pleasant surprise. After you practice Power Yoga for a month or so, your response is likely to be much quieter: You may stop and take a deep breath, clear your mind, and — AHA! — remember right where you left them. Ah, the power of the Power Yoga practice.

 When you're relaxed, you tend to be more self-confident and hold a positive outlook. Most of us spend a lot of time thinking about things that we've done wrong or could have done better, worrying about things that we're afraid we'll do wrong (or forget to do altogether), and just plain beating up on ourselves. Feeding your body and mind with proper relaxation encourages you to toss those self-defeating thoughts aside and feel good about yourself. Life is way more fun when it's upbeat and positive!

Relaxation also helps to heal the body. Stress weakens your body and makes you more susceptible to illness, injury, and disease. In fact, stress is closely linked to heart disease, one of the major causes of death in the United States today. By helping you to relieve tension and avoid stress, you can think of relaxation as good medicine for your body. Relaxation exercises have even been found to lower blood pressure. Combine the benefits of relaxation with the wonderful exercise you get in every Power Yoga session, and you're giving your heart a powerful gift!

Are you sleeping?

The deep relaxation you feel in Power Yoga is similar to a state of sleep, but you stay awake and very aware; that awareness is what makes deep relaxation so powerful. When you sleep, you close your eyes and (with luck) drift off, pass through a dream phase, then awaken when you're rested. Unfortunately, you may often have a hard time falling asleep, feeling restless, or having your sleep interrupted, and get up in the morning feeling as if you haven't slept at all. On the other hand, when you do a Deep Relaxation Exercise in your Power Yoga routine, you play a more active role in the relaxation process (as odd as that may sound). During Deep Relaxation, you physically and mentally target each area of your body for relaxation, incorporate self-hypnosis to make sure your body and mind really unwind, and you regenerate positive thought and self-confidence. During Deep Relaxation, you never really turn off the power completely — but you certainly slow it down a lot. And it feels great to get back some of the energy you burn running around trying to keep up with daily life.

Practicing your deep relaxation techniques

No matter what kind of Yoga you practice — hard, soft, or any variety in between — always end your session with deep relaxation. In fact, knowing that a wonderful relaxation session is yet to come can help get you through the most challenging workout!

The Corpse (or Sponge) Pose is the one most commonly used in deep relaxation exercises. The Sanskrit name for this pose is *savasana.* The word *sava* means "corpse or dead body" and *asana,* of course, means "pose." When practicing *savasana,* you lie completely motionless on your back. If you don't find the thought of being a corpse very relaxing, you can think of yourself as a sponge soaking up energy from the universe.

Striking a relaxing yet powerful pose

Power Yoga offers a number of poses perfect for relaxing or meditating: They're comfortable, calming, and easy to do. Try them all and see what feels comfortable to you. Check out Chapter 8 for more detail about each sitting posture.

✔ **The Corpse:** Lay down on your back with your legs extended and your feet about one foot apart; extend your arms by your sides with palms facing upward. (If you have lower back problems you can put a pillow under your knees for support.) Close your eyes, clear your mind, and begin your slow deep breathing. Starting with your feet and working up to the top of your body, tense and relax each muscle, one at a time. When you reach your scalp, go back over your body once again; finish by suggesting that your mind relax completely (see the Cheat Sheet).

✔ **Easy Posture:** Sit in a regular cross-legged position (refer to Figure 8-2). If your feet start to fall asleep separate them so your legs don't push on your ankles.

✔ **Half Lotus:** Sit with one ankle resting on top of the opposite hip or leg. The other leg is bent and comfortable, resting on the floor, as you sit cross-legged. (Refer to Figure 8-7.)

✔ **Lotus:** Sit with your ankles folded onto opposite hips (refer to Figure 8-10).

✔ **Thunderbolt:** Sit on your heels (refer to Figure 8-5). You can sit between your heels if your knees don't mind.

The Deep Relaxation exercise is an essential "cap" to every Power Yoga session. If you need a gentle reminder of the Deep Relaxation process, you can return to the "Persuading Trainer Exercise," in Chapter 8.

Sitting and breathing in the Easy Posture

Before you go into your deep relaxation, you should slow yourself down with some yogic breathing techniques. This breathing exercise can help you relax completely as you move into the deep relaxation phase of the workout.

Being calm and centered during your breathing exercise is essential. Quiet your mind, and make yourself as comfortable as possible — while maintaining good posture, of course! As always, you can sit on a small pillow or in a chair if you find that more comfortable than the floor.

Follow these steps to easy breathing:

1. **Extend your arms over your knees, resting your wrists on your knees, with your palms facing upward; form *Jnana Mudra* with your hands (see the Cheat Sheet).**

2. **Begin breathing slowly, taking in and expelling as much oxygen as you can.**

3. **Take 10–15 slow, deep breaths.**

4. **Lie back into the Corpse Pose and move to the deep relaxation exercise.**

Relax, why don't you?

As luxurious as deep relaxation feels, don't think of it as a "luxury" add-on to your Power Yoga practice. The deep relaxation exercise is one of the most important parts of your whole Power Yoga routine. Make sure you wrap up every Power Yoga practice with a deep relaxation exercise, or your body, mind, *and* practice will suffer. You and I both live in a fast paced society, and we can't avoid absorbing lots of stress and anxiety in our daily lives. A good, fast-paced Power Yoga workout helps to melt the effects of that tension from our muscles, but we need the relaxation phase of the workout to wash the effects of that tension from our minds. Deep relaxation is one of the simple things in life that mean a lot. So don't overlook this opportunity for a mini-vacation at the end of every Power Yoga session!

Enjoying deep relaxation in the Corpse Posture (Savasana)

The Sanskrit word *sava* means "corpse." In this posture, you lie flat on the floor, completely relaxed and motionless. The Corpse Posture, shown in Figure 14-1, is a great way to experience the deep relaxation phase that caps off your Power Yoga session.

In the deep relaxation phase, you will release stress and tension throughout your entire body and mind. Your blood pressure decreases, your heart rate slows, and you are rewarded with an euphoric feeling that can last for hours. You also will relieve stress and tension, and create total relaxation in every fiber of your body. The deep relaxation phase promotes complete physical and mental rejuvenation as it boosts your motivation and self-esteem.

Figure 14-1:
To get the most from the Corpse Posture, pay close attention to your Yoga breathing techniques.

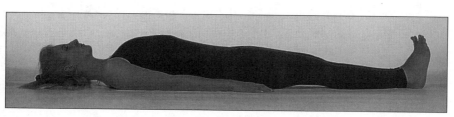

1. Lie on your back, with your arms at your sides and your legs extended.

   This is called the Corpse Pose.

2. Close your eyes, relax, and begin taking slow, deep breaths.

3. Lift your right leg about 12 inches from the floor, tense every muscle in your leg for a few seconds, relax, and then gently lower your leg to the floor; repeat this step with your left leg.

4. Tighten the muscles in your hips and buttocks for a few seconds, and then relax and let your gluteus muscles "melt" into the floor.

5. Arch your back, pressing down with your elbows and shoulders as you expand your chest toward the ceiling; hold this position for a few seconds, and then relax, lowering your back to the floor.

6. Press your lower back into the floor by tightening your buttock and stomach muscles as you press against the floor; hold this position for a few seconds, and then relax completely.

7. Lift your right arm about 12 inches off the floor, tensing all the muscles; hold this position for a few seconds, and then relax and lower your arm to the floor; repeat this step using your left arm.

8. Roll your head slowly to the right, and then to the left; return your head to the center, and relax.

9. Fill your mouth with air, blowing your cheeks out like balloons; hold for a couple of seconds, and then relax and release the air.

10. Gently stretch all your facial muscles, and then relax them.

11. Close your eyes, take 5 slow, deep breaths, and clear your mind.

12. Working from your toes to your head, visualize each part of your body and tell each muscle to relax.

13. Visualize your heart, and mentally ask your heart to relax.

14. Visualize your brain, and calm it by releasing your thoughts.

15. Clear your mind of all but the most pleasant and positive thoughts.

16. After 5–30 minutes, slowly stretch your arms over your head on an inhalation and then roll over onto your right side, with your arms and legs slightly bent; remain in this position for a few breaths.

17. Gradually return to a sitting position and try to preserve the positive, uplifting thoughts you created.

During your deep relaxation, you are cultivating your sacred space and watering the beautiful garden inside of you. There is a peaceful place within you that you can find when you quiet the chatter in your mind. It is in this sacred place that you are free of stress and tension and your mind is clear. When you cultivate this sacred place during relaxation, you are cleaning the path to it, sweeping the steps and making it easier to find. In time, you will be able to find your way to your sacred place whenever you need it. Anytime you are faced with a stressful situation, you can go to that space and relax. Anytime you are faced with a difficult decision, you can go to that space and find clarity. So take time to cultivate that garden everyday.

Discovering the Power of Meditation

Before I delve into the benefits of meditation, let me give you a poetic taste of what I feel about it:

> *Travel the journey within*
>
> *The quiet mind seeks the power of the whole universe*
>
> *The whole universe seeks the tranquility of the quiet mind*
>
> *Be still and the all will embrace you*

Meditation is an ancient practice that's part of many cultures and religions. Meditation helps you gain control over your restless mind; you gain focus, peace, and mental rejuvenation. Meditation can greatly enhance your Power Yoga practice by bringing you better concentration, mental organization, and increased self-confidence.

Mediation in some shape or form exists in most major religions, including Christianity. Each person has a unique approach to using meditation to enhance his or her own path, and different meditation practices are taught by different religious groups.

The American Indian healers that we call *shamans* entered meditative states that lasted for hours — even days — through drumming, chanting, dancing, and ingesting or smoking hallucinogenic plants. Other groups enter meditative states through prayer or contemplation of the divine.

Meditation is a popular technique among Buddhists and was used by Buddha himself. After Buddha had practiced a restrictive diet, simplicity of lifestyle, and Yoga for many years, he felt he had looked everywhere for enlightenment; then — as the legend goes — he decided to look inward and observe his mind for seven straight days and nights. He went into deep meditation, and when he emerged from his meditative state he understood the nature of our existence and therefore was named The Awakened One *(Buddha)*.

Who's meditating today? Some years ago, people associated meditation with monks, nuns, sages, and Yoga teachers; today, people in all walks of life are meditating — the milkman, the garbage collector, the dishwasher, the professional athlete, the attorney, and of course, those Hollywood stars! Anyone and everyone who wants to improve the quality of his or her mind and life is trying meditation. (For a complete run-down on meditation, check out *Meditation For Dummies* by Stephen Bodian (Hungry Minds, Inc.).

Sitting still

One of the benefits of Yoga is to help people who meditate sit still for hours. Sitting is hard on the hips and the back. Your Power Yoga practice helps open up your hips, so sitting isn't as difficult as it used to be. Even so, you may want to lengthen your meditation or relaxation sessions gradually to give your body a chance to become accustomed to sitting in stillness. You can also try sitting on a blanket or a meditation cushion. Elevating your hips above your ankles helps relieve a little tension in your hips. Trust me, it gets easier as you keep practicing.

Combining meditation and Power Yoga

You may be a little confused about what meditation has to do with Power Yoga. Well, Yoga was originally created as a tool for enlightenment or self-realization. The masters who developed Yoga sought inner peace and knowledge by studying and disciplining their physical bodies, and by being in touch with nature. Just like meditation, Power Yoga helps you bring your mind to stillness In a lot of ways, it's easier to quiet the mind through Yoga *asanas* because they take a lot of mental concentration. At the end of your practice you usually feel free of stress. It's a good time to sit in meditation, especially if you have a hard time calming and focusing your mind.

You can think of meditation as mental exercise, to get your mind in shape. After you try it a couple of times, you'll understand that it takes real power to quiet your mind.

Finding your meditation style

When you first start meditating, you may try several different approaches until you find the one that really clicks for you. The following are some meditation techniques you can try. Remember this is your personal journey, so you want to find what method works best for you. So strike a pose — a seated pose, that is — and test-drive a meditation technique or two:

- ✔ **Chant:** Almost all religions use chanting or singing as a means of clearing the mind and connecting to the power of the universe. If you don't know any traditional chants about God or gods, saints or sages, you can make up you own, listen to recorded chanting or any relaxing music, for that matter (see the "Meditating Music" sidebar for some of my personal favorites).

✔ **Concentrate on your breath:** You can begin a meditation session or a Power Yoga session by focusing on your breath. Focusing on your breathing can clear your mind and get you ready for meditation or practice. A useful technique for beginners is to count breaths. You may want to try counting backwards to make it a little more challenging, and to focus your attention on what you're doing.

✔ **Gaze at a photo, drawing, or image:** Gazing at an image without thinking is a fun meditation technique; if the picture happens to be of a saint or sage, you may find that gazing helps you make a spiritual connection. You can also try staring at a candle flame. If you don't have a candle, you can always gaze at the cover of this book.

✔ **Reflect on sacred writings:** You can read a passage from the Bible, the *Bhagavad-Gita*, the Koran, a new-age spiritual book, or any writing that you find inspiring. Then sit quietly and let the words sink in. You don't need to analyze the words, just be still and let their meaning sink into your heart.

✔ **Repeat a meaningful word or saying:** Many people like to meditate on the word OM (pronounced aum), which symbolizes your connection to the universe. You may want to start your own mantra by repeating a simple phrase to help bring you to a meditative state; any phrase that speaks to you will do — something like "Health is Wealth" or "Kindness speaks through its action." You may want to concentrate on something you want to manifest in your life. (Maybe the phrase, "Strength through softness," works for you?)

✔ **Visualize a shape or an object or a color:** Many people begin meditation by visualizing a purple circle, or a red square. Focus on the color and shape of any object and allow your other thoughts to float away. Visualization can give your mind a focal point and help you to still the chatter in your head.

✔ **Visualize yourself in nature:** One of my favorite techniques is to picture yourself lying in a field or on a beach, in a beautiful, natural place. You stare up at the clouds and every time a thought comes into your head, you see that thought on a cloud. Then you watch the cloud float out of your mind, out of the sky. Gradually, you see fewer and fewer clouds and have fewer and fewer thoughts.

Meditating music

The following discs can help you to still the chatter and set the mood for your meditation practice.

- **The Harmonic Vibrations of Crystal Singing Bowls** by Crystal Voices. This CD is composed of the unique and relaxing sounds of crystal singing bowls combined with voice, chimes, and running water. It includes a guided meditation to clear the energy centers (known as "Chakras") in the body.

- **Higher Ground** by Steven Halpern. This CD provides a slow and steady sound designed to help you relax completely. (www.stevenhalpern.com)

- **Live on Earth** by Krishna Das. If you want to start chanting, this is a fun, energetic CD. Kirtan-style chanting is done in call and response fashion so the singer sings the words and the crowd repeats it back. The words and some explanations are included in the sleeve. (www.krishnadas.com).

- **Waking the Cobra** by Baird Hersey. This CD features overtone chanting in which the voice produces a unique higher tone. The slow meditative chanting is perfect for meditation and it also includes pieces to help clear the energy centers of the body. (www.waking-the-cobra.com)

Part IV
Focusing on Specific Areas

The 5th Wave   By Rich Tennant

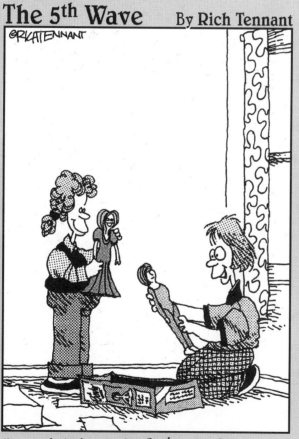

"...and this one's Yogini Barbie. She doesn't come with a lot of stuff, but you can bend her into 13 different positions without anything breaking."

In this part . . .

Want to increase your endurance, become more flexible, build up your muscles and your strength? All of the above? You're in the right part. I give you separate chapters and specific routines so that you can target a particular area. You can, of course, combine the exercises in all these chapters and become your own Wonder Woman or Superman.

Chapter 15

Bending Like Gumby: A Flexibility Workout

*W*hat would you give to maintain the physical flexibility of youth through your entire life? Well, it's entirely possible that you can. We're all born with a relatively flexible body; but as time goes on our muscles get tight and our joints start to ache. We become less and less active and, as a result, even less flexible. Of course, your own progression through this uncomfortable cycle depends on how physically active you are and what physical activities you engage in. As rule, though, men tend to be less flexible than women.

I named this chapter after the cartoon character Gumby out of deep yogic respect for his ultimate flexibility. In this chapter, I give you sound advice for building your own flexibility (and you don't have to turn green or spend all day with Pokey, the orange horse). I share some of my favorite stretching exercises and show you how to incorporate flexibility training into your Power Yoga schedule, how to know — and respect — your limits, and how to avoid stretch-related injuries. And, of course, I finish up by giving you a Power Yoga routine packed with postures and exercises specifically targeted to increase your flexibility.

There's no reason to get all bent out of shape about any lack of flexibility — just read on, and get ready to "go Gumby" with me!

Playing it Safe as You Stretch

Flexibility makes you stronger and less prone to injury. Think about it — a rubber band stretches a lot further than a piece of string. When you lengthen your muscles through stretching exercises, you make them much more capable of withstanding pressure and resisting damage. Flexibility can help you in countless ways as you move through your daily routines. Whether you're climbing in and out of your car, or climbing on the roof of your house to clean the gutters, your flexibility helps you remain strong, stable, and balanced, so you avoid twisting, slipping, and stumbling your way through life.

As you incorporate stretching exercises into your Yoga practice, you should know how to safely "play your edge." Now, I'm not talking about knowing the right time to sell your stocks and make a financial killing. I'm talking about gauging just how far your muscles can stretch without being damaged. Think of your Power Yoga edge as the edge of a cliff. When you walk up to the edge of a cliff, you can enjoy a beautiful view; a step too far, though, and that view gets obscured by the pain of your fall.

In Power Yoga, your workouts should take you to the edge of your "capability cliff"; that's how you get the marvelous benefit of building your strength, balance, endurance, and flexibility. But if you take your workout too far, you can seriously injure yourself and ruin the Power Yoga experience for some time to come. And nowhere is this warning truer than as it applies to stretching your muscles.

Stretching is the key to building flexibility. Ideally, you want to walk the edge in your Power Yoga stretching exercises in order to make real progress in improving your flexibility. In each *asana* (pose), stretch as far as you comfortably can, then relax, maintain your Yoga breathing, and slowly back off from the stretch. As your practice progresses, you should be able to take your stretches further — safely extending your edge for ever greater benefits. Dance on the edge, enjoy the view, and expand your flexibility gradually, over a period of time. And always listen to your body and respect its limits to avoid injuries.

Following are some tips for playing your Power Yoga edge safely:

- **Practice in a warm environment:** Your body is more flexible and supple when it's warm, and the warmth helps protect your muscles from injury.

- **Push to where you feel the stretch, then relax in that area:** After a week or so, try to slowly expand your stretch. If your muscles are noticeably sore more than a day after your stretching workout, back off for a few days and then try again.

- **Remember that you're the only one who knows how far to stretch your body:** If you're working with a teacher or partner, make sure to let him or her know when you reach the end of your "comfortable" stretch.

Interpreting your body's pain messages

Lots of people don't think of Yoga as a form of fitness training. But if you're practicing Power Yoga, you understand how physically demanding it can be. As with any kind of athletic activity, a high-energy Power Yoga workout may leave you with a few minor muscle twinges now and then. When you teach your body new skills or challenge your muscles, you can expect occasional, minor pain. But really bad pain or pain that lasts more than a day or so isn't a twinge — it's a warning.

If you experience repeated or persistent pain in one area of your body and it doesn't seem to go away, don't shrug it off; your body is telling you to stop doing something that's injuring it. If you have this kind of pain, you need to determine what part of your activity (whether it's part of your Power Yoga routine or not) is causing the pain; then, you need to scale back that activity, change the way you're doing it, or avoid it altogether.

Yoga-related injuries are often the result of over-stretching. Cross-training — incorporating other activities in addition to Power Yoga into your schedule — is one of the best ways to avoid these types of injuries. And make sure that you begin any hard physical activity with a slow warm-up, and end it with a cool-down exercise. Your muscles don't want to develop "whiplash" as you jolt them in and out of high-power action.

Your Power Yoga breathing and deep relaxation techniques are important tools for safeguarding your muscles from injury, too — don't ever bypass them in your practice. And of course, never forget Buddha's advice to "follow the middle line." Moderation is the key to a healthy life, safe fitness, and an effective Power Yoga practice.

Keep these tips in mind when you're translating those messages from your body:

- ✔ Sore muscles are a natural part of getting in shape, as long as the soreness goes away in a few days.

- ✔ The Power Yoga system works like this: Work your body, stretch your muscles, and *always* rest and relax your body.

- ✔ Determine the difference between being lazy and being tired. Often, a lack of exercise makes you feel tired and run down. Follow your Power Yoga practice with commitment, but use moderation.

Your level of flexibility depends on how tight your muscles are and how much you practice your Power Yoga. If you aren't fully flexible, and you try to fold in half or stretch your body in some other dramatic way, look out! You're going to hurt tomorrow. In Power Yoga, you discover that over-stretching won't make you flexible any faster; it just makes you sore. Power Yoga delivers some easy-to-remember lessons in patience. And that patience stays with you as you leave the studio for work, home, or other activities. Standing in line, traffic jams, and flight delays won't stress you out: You get there when you get there. You always do, and you always have. But you'll realize that your journey wasn't as peaceful before you learned the patience that accompanies a Power Yoga lifestyle.

Stretching your flexibility training

You may as well be prepared for it: One of these days, you'll hit a wall in your Power Yoga flexibility training. You'll feel like you can't progress anymore and that you'll have to live with your current level of flexibility. But don't give into this feeling; your quickest path to flexibility is to follow that old saying, "Take two steps back to go one step forward."

The chances are good that when you feel stalled it's because you're trying to go too far, too quickly. Take a few days off from your practice, use an easier routine, or go back to beginner-level stretches for a while. When you start progressing again, you're likely to find that you can go much further than before.

Some other ideas for safely building your flexibility over time are:

- **Counter-stretch:** Always balance your flexibility training across your body. Stretch the muscles on both sides of your leg — and in both legs. If you stretch your stomach, stretch your back. Counter-stretching stabilizes your body's strength and helps you build flexibility without injury.

- **Move smoothly into and out of each stretch:** All Power Yoga movements should flow in one smooth, gentle, rhythm, but stretching exercises really demand fluid transitions. Don't jerk into a stretch, and never try to use a "bounce" to get just a little bit further than your muscles want to go. Keep all of your stretching motions calm, gentle, and controlled.

- **Concentrate on your breathing:** When you're working out, it's easy to forget about your breathing, but it's also a big mistake. Deep inhalations help speed oxygen into your bloodstream and muscle tissue, making all of your movements easier. Deep exhalations help you sink deeper into long stretches. And slow regular breathing keeps your mind calm and focused, so it does a better job of directing your muscular activity.

- **Pay attention to the area you're stretching:** As you move into a stretch, focus on the muscles you're stretching. Cultivate a mind-body connection and visualize yourself achieving greater flexibility in that area. By using the power of your mind to focus your body's work, you get the maximum benefit from every posture.

- **Make stretching exercises an ongoing part of your routine:** Don't try to cram all of your stretching exercise into one day of the week. And be sure to work the areas where you need it most. Don't be lulled into repeating Yoga postures that require the least effort on your part. Work on the areas of your body — and your Power Yoga practice — that need the most work.

Power Routine for Stretching Your Flexibility

I talk about the whys, hows, wheres, and whens of flexibility training throughout this chapter (and this book). Table 15-1 outlines a way to put all that good advice (and those powerful postures) to work in a full-fledged Power Yoga routine. This routine can help extend the flexibility of your entire body, and it's a great addition to your list of Power Yoga routines.

And don't forget to think of this as just that — an *addition* to your other Power Yoga routines. To keep your Power Yoga training balanced and effective, don't forget to alternate this routine with a basic routine from Chapter 11, 12, or 13 (whichever is most appropriate for your level of practice).

So, get your partner and your props, move to a warm room (take this book!), start your slow, deep, Yoga breathing, then take your time as you work through this routine. I think you'll really enjoy it, and I know it will improve your flexibility. Good luck, Gumby!

Table 15-1	Flexibility Power Routine	
Exercise	*Duration*	*Reference*
Yoga Breathing	10–20 breaths	Cheat Sheet
Seated Forward Bend	5 breaths	Figure 11-4a
Expanded Seated Forward Bend	5 breaths/3 repetitions	Figure 11-4b
Doug's Favorite Leg Split	5 breaths/2 repetitions	Figure 15-1
Extended Foot One Leg Stand with partner	5 breaths each side	Figure 7-2, 7-3
Cobra	5 breaths/2 repetitions	Figure 10-3a
Bridge	5 breaths/2 repetitions	Figure 13-10
Wheel	5 breaths/2 repetitions	Figure 13-8b
Downward Facing Dog	5 breaths	Cheat Sheet
Persuading Posture Trainer	5 breaths	Figure 8-3
Spine Toner	5 breaths	Figure 9-1
Moonbeam Bird	5 breaths each side	Figure 15-2
Windmill	2 repetitions on each side	Figure 9-11
Breathing and deep relaxation	5–15 minutes	Figure 14-1

At the end of your workout, don't forget to spend at least 5–10 minutes relaxing in the Corpse position doing a Yoga breathing exercise. Then, take a moment to congratulate yourself, Gumby — you've started stretching your flexibility limits!

Presenting Power Postures for Your Inner Gumby

Almost every Power Yoga exercise and routine in this book can improve your flexibility — after all, flexibility training is central to the whole Power Yoga thing. But in this chapter, I want to show you a few of my favorite postures that really zero in on giving your muscles a strong, powerful stretching workout. The postures in this section are new flexibility ones included in the flexibility routine I offer in Table 15-1.

Doug's Favorite Leg Split (Hanumanasana)

This posture is known in the United States as the Leg Split, but in the Hindu culture its name is *Hanumanasana*. In the Sanskrit language, *Hanuman* is a monkey god, famous for making giant leaps over the ocean. In this Yoga posture you make like Hanuman, as you split your legs for that great leap over the hurdle of limited flexibility.

Practicing the Leg Split tones and strengthens your leg muscles, stretches out your lower back, and expands your chest. This is an excellent posture for runners to help lengthen tight muscles. A word of advice for anyone with limited flexibility: Have a pillow or bolster handy to use as a prop during this exercise.

1. **From the Downward Facing Dog posture (see the Cheat Sheet) step forward with your right foot and place it between your hands, and lower your left knee to the floor behind you for support.**

   Support your torso with your arms and try to square your hips with your extended right leg.

   If you need support, place a bolster or block under the hamstring muscle of your right thigh (see Figure 15-1a) to make this exercise more comfortable. As your balance improves, you can extend your arms up, as the yogis in the photos do (the b-side yogi is yours truly).

2. **Split your legs as far as you can comfortably stretch, by extending your right leg forward and your left leg backward.**

This is where the bolster comes in handy, as you allow the weight of your torso to rest on the bolster. If you aren't using a bolster, you can use your hands to give you some extra support.

3. **Keep your hips, shoulders and torso facing forward toward your extended right leg. Hold this position for 5 slow deep breaths.**

   Figure 15-1b shows the advanced Full Leg Split, without props.

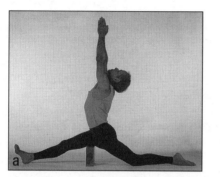

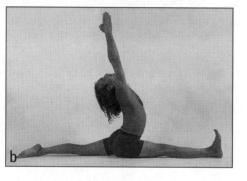

Figure 15-1:
Using a
pillow or
bolster as
support (a)
helps make
the Leg Split
(b) more
comfortable.

4. **Slowly push down with your hands, lift your hips, and bend your right knee, as you step your right foot back and return to the Downward Facing Dog position.**

5. **Repeat these steps, extending your left leg forward in Step 1.**

Flying with the Moonbeam Bird (Chakorasana)

The Sanskrit word *chakora* is the name of a beautiful bird from Hindu legend; the Chakora was said to feed on moonbeams. This Yoga posture is difficult, but like that legendary bird, it's very beautiful, too. This *asana* stretches out your hamstrings, opens your hips, and strengthens abdominals and arms.

The Chakorasana also teaches balance and coordination, so it's a good posture for building your self-confidence, too. Follow these steps to fly with the Moonbeam Bird:

1. **Start from a Seated Angle Position (see the Cheat Sheet).**

2. **Bend your left knee, and place your left foot on your right thigh as if you were preparing for the Lotus Posture (refer to Figure 8-10).**

   Cradle your left leg with your arms, bending your arms and lifting your left leg up, holding it to your body like a baby.

3. **Try to bring your leg all the way up to your shoulders, pulling your leg in toward your chest and keeping your knee bent.**

   This movement is included here to open your hips, to better prepare you for the rest of this posture.

4. **Try to put your left arm under your left leg: Grasp your left ankle with both hands, tilt your head forward, keep your knees slightly bent, push the leg back behind your head, and hook it behind your neck.**

   As you lift your leg higher, try to place your left leg all the way up onto your left shoulder.

5. **If you have trouble getting your leg to move below your head to your neck, push your head backward slightly to push the leg back behind you.**

   After your leg is behind your head, push with your left shoulder slightly in a circular motion to get the leg back behind you a little further.

6. **Place both hands palm down on the floor beside your hips; push down into the floor, straightening your arms as you lift your hips off the floor with your leg behind your head.**

   Hold this position for five very slow, deep breaths (see Figure 15-2).

7. **After the fifth exhalation, bend your elbows and gently lower your hips.**

8. **Lift your hands, move your leg from behind your head, and lower it to the floor.**

9. **Return to the Seated Angle position.**

10. **Repeat Steps 2 through 9, this time bending your right knee and placing your right leg back behind your head.**

11. **When you finish, relax into the Seated Angle Pose.**

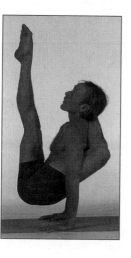

Figure 15-2:
The legendary Moonbeam Bird feeds on moonbeams. As you practice this Yoga posture, you gaze up as though you're looking at the moon.

A good counter-stretch for this exercise is the Bridge Posture (refer to Figure 13-10), which works the muscles on the front of your leg.

Flexibility Training with a Partner

Another really good way to improve your flexibility is to practice with a partner. A partner can help you help you move into a stretch and lengthen your body within the stretch. Partner work is especially helpful when you're just beginning a Power Yoga practice and your body is still quite stiff. I cover working with a partner in Chapter 22, but I offer one flexibility exercise here.

Working in tandem

Your partner can help you maintain the right alignment within Yoga postures as you stretch. And partner work is a lot of fun; you get to exchange energy with your partner during a workout, and you learn a lot by helping your partner work through Yoga *asanas* and exercises. Power Yoga offers a lot of really great partner exercises. In fact, I devote a whole chapter to them later in this book — see Chapter 22.

As in other areas of life, though, a Power Yoga partnership is only as good as the communication that goes into it. Partner work is great only as long as you communicate your capabilities and limitations to your partner. You have to be the pilot of your own ship: You tell your partner when you want help to do more — and when you've gone as far as you can.

Stretcher's Choice: Extended Foot One Leg Stand (Uttihita Hasta Padangusthasana)

This exercise is one of Gumby's personal favorite partner stretches. Quick, go grab your partner and get ready to stretch your Power Yoga relationship to a whole new level.

You may recognize this little gem as a variation on one in Chapter 7 — Extended Foot One Leg Stand. The posture I show you here, though, adds the wonderful element of working with a Power Yoga partner. In this posture, your partner helps you extend as comfortably as you can into the leg stretch. But don't forget to let your partner know just how far you want to stretch.

1. **Stand with your back to a wall facing your partner who stands about two feet away from you.**

2. **Follow the instructions for the Extended Foot One Leg Stand in Chapter 7 — Figure 7-3 shows you how to do this by yourself — but let your partner carry your leg through the stretch, giving you a little stretch extension.**

Chapter 16

Taking on Xena and Hercules: Strengthening Postures

*W*hen I say "strength," any number of things may come to mind. But I'm not referring to your strength of character, nor to your breath after you've downed a big slice of garlic bread. Nope, in this chapter, I talk to you about ways you can build your *body* strength by practicing Power Yoga. Power Yoga is one of the most effective ways I've found to build powerful, whole-body, muscular strength. Zena and Hercules were famous for their incredible strength. If you've ever dreamed of developing that kind of muscle-power, this chapter is your ticket to Mount Olympus!

In this chapter, I share some good information with you about how to approach the strength-building phase of your Power Yoga practice. I talk about pacing yourself in full-power workouts, the importance of cross-training, and the pros and cons of using energy-boosting diet supplements. I show you poses you can incorporate into any Power Yoga routine to boost its strength-building benefits. And I wrap things up by outlining a Power Yoga workout fit for any superhero. So get going, and soon you'll unleash the inner Zena or Hercules that lies within that Power Yoga body of yours!

Putting the Muscle to Your Workouts

Many people think of Yoga as a good way to build flexibility and a nice relaxation technique. Of course, Power Yoga adds the benefits of increasing your endurance and helping you stay fit and trim. But any student of Power Yoga can tell you that their practice is as much about gaining strength as it is about any of these other benefits.

Yes, Virginia, you can build enormous amounts of strength through your Power Yoga practice. But if you're serious about "pumping up" with Power Yoga, you need to approach your practice with a warrior's commitment. So, before you hit the Yoga mat, take a minute to read through some of the strength-building basics of the Power Yoga practice.

Slow down, Herc — Rome wasn't built in a day

From the solid blocks of the Great Pyramids of Egypt to the green canopy of the Brazilian rain forest, great things take a long time to build or grow. If you want a great body, plan on spending some time developing it. Power Yoga is a powerful tool for pumping up, but you get the best results by gradually building your muscle strength through regular practice and periodic rest.

Move slowly and let your body adjust on a daily basis. After a period of two weeks to a month of regular Power Yoga practice, you should notice definite improvements in your strength. Don't let that bulging bicep encourage you to go wild in your Power Yoga workouts, though. Just keep gradually building your strength by varying the difficulty, length, and exercise repetitions in your practice. And don't forget to take an occasional rest. If you give your body a break now and then, you find that you progress much faster — and go farther — in your fitness improvements.

I remember very vividly my first experience with Ashtanga Yoga (the mother of Power Yoga). My brother and I, two hot-shot Yoga-surfers from Texas, had been practicing a fair amount of traditional Yoga consistently for about six years. We thought we were in great shape — and quite strong. That is, until we walked into David Williams and Nancy Gilgoff's Ashtanga Yoga class in Southern California. To put it bluntly, the workout we got that day made us very humble; my brother and I quickly realized that we were a long way from being as strong as we could be.

But we were hooked, and started practicing Ashtanga Yoga almost every day. Our teachers urged us to back off a bit and take some rest days, but we didn't listen. "Resting is non-productive," we thought, so we kept busting it every day, ignoring our sore muscles and shrugging off our exhaustion.

Well, only a few months later we realized we had hit the wall; we weren't progressing at all. So, as much as we hated to do it, we started to take some rest days and lightened up our practice for a while. Much to our surprise, our sore muscles disappeared over the next few weeks, and in a few more weeks we found ourselves much stronger than before. The moral of this story is that you should always listen to your body.

Building strength for today and everyday

You don't have to be a superhero, Greek god, or the Governor of Minnesota to benefit from building your muscle strength. Strong muscles help you out in many everyday activities, from lifting your kids, working on your house, or playing a fast game of tennis. And, as you age, the benefits of strong muscles become even more important. Strong people are less likely to lose their balance and fall; and good muscle strength builds confidence, coordination, and a positive, healthy attitude toward life. Your Power Yoga practice will build your muscles, just as the daily practice of weightlifters, dancers, and rock-climbers boosts their strength. But don't be impatient. You aren't on a fitness "clock." Commit to a regular practice schedule, and watch your body gradually gain strength over the weeks and months ahead.

You don't gain from pain, so don't just do it!

When you first start doing a lot of strengthening poses in Power Yoga, you're likely to have sore muscles. Don't think you should just "work through" this pain and keep driving on. If you don't let your body recuperate and *slowly* build strength, you'll never make any real strength or fitness progress. So, when a Power Yoga workout leaves you sore, you should back off the next day, do some light Power Yoga training or cross-training, and then come back another day to try those muscle-building poses again.

And don't ever forget that it's much easier to avoid injuries than to overcome them. So, if you feel pain from doing strenuous, strengthening Yoga exercises, and that pain lasts more than a day or two, you really need to back off and give your body a rest. Take some days off from exercise — lie back in a hammock and drink some lemonade or curl up on the sofa and read a book. Even a light walk will give your body a restful break from hard exercise. Again, if you let your body be your guide, you can't take a wrong turn on the path to fitness.

Keep on cross-training!

If you want to progress and gain strength in your Power Yoga practice, try to cross-train with other Yoga routines and non-Yogic exercises. Balance is the name of the game in Yoga, and cross-training is the best way to balance your body's development. If you are doing strengthening poses one week, maybe the next week try some flexibility poses or endurance routines. Make sure the exercises and postures in your routines work to strengthen your legs, arms, butt, stomach, and back, as well as your heart and lungs. Varying your Power Yoga routines — the exercises and sequencing of postures in every workout — is important for maintaining a balanced, whole-body strengthening program.

Muscling into Your Xena and Hercules Power Yoga Routine

And now for the real powerhouse — a Power Yoga routine designed for maximum muscle-ocity. If this routine doesn't convince you that Yoga can definitely be a strengthening exercise, I'll eat my Yoga mat. In fact, this routine may be harder than any exercise workout you've ever tried before. But with perseverance and patience, it can be your powerful ticket to whole-body strength.

Table 16-1 lists the Power Yoga exercises included in this routine. The table also lists the number of repetitions for each exercise and the chapter (and figure numbers) in which the exercise is fully described. Take your time to familiarize yourself with this routine, then go for it!

Table 16-1	Strength Routine	
Exercise	*Duration*	*Reference*
Mother Lode Salutation	10 repetitions	Figures 10-1a, 10-9, 10-5, 10-8, 10-3b, 10-9, 10-10
Warrior II	5 breaths each side	figure 12-4
Downward Dog Push-Ups	10 repetitions	Figure 12-1
Seated Forward Bend	5 breaths/2 repetitions	Figure 11-4
Bridge	5 breaths/2repetitions	Figure 13-10
Wheel or Bridge	5 breaths/2 repetitions	Figures 13-8 & 13-10
Boat to Scale	5 breaths/5repetitions	Figures 11-6 & 12-12
Crane and Running Man	5 breaths/2repetitions	Figures 16-1 & 16-2
Yoga Breathing	20–30 breaths	Cheat Sheet
Relaxation	5–15 minutes	Figure 14-1

This Power Yoga routine is based on strengthening exercises, so it isn't a completely balanced routine to use as your only Yoga routine. These exercises are great strength-builders, but they're only effective as part of a balanced exercise program of other Power Yoga routines and cross-training activities.

Let the Games Begin

Okay, future Power Yoga Olympians, it's time to try out some of my favorite strength-building Yoga poses. The exercises I show you in this section should dismiss any questions you may have about whether or not Power Yoga is tough enough to buff you up. Incorporating these postures into your Power Yoga routines is a sure way to build muscle strength.

Think about it this way: weightlifting is a tried-and-true method for pumping up your muscles, right? Well, in almost every Power Yoga exercise, you're actually lifting weight — the weight of your own body. You lift, pull, push, and balance your body's weight, and, as a result, incorporate important anaerobic exercise into your Power Yoga workout. *Anaerobic exercises* are muscle-strengthening powerhouses; combining this exercise element with your flexibility training gives you some of the most intense fitness benefits to be found in any exercise program. The poses in this section are strong anaerobic contenders in the Power Yoga practice Hall of Fame. (*Anaerobic exercise* involves the strengthening of specific muscles, without involving strong respiratory workout. These exercises usually take only a few seconds to complete.)

Pumping it up with Crane and Running Man (Bakasana)

In Sanskrit, the word *baka* means "crane." In the initial variation of this posture, you resemble a crane wading in a pond. In the Running Man variation on this pose, you resemble Arnold (pronounced Ah-nold) running and flexing his muscles in the movie *The Running Man*.

The Crane and its partner Running Man are both great for building your stomach, arm, and shoulder muscles. These postures also strengthen your wrists and improve your balance. The Crane pose is hard to master; it takes balance, strength, and technique.

1. **Start from the Downward Facing Dog position (see the Cheat Sheet or Figure 10-3b), then bend your elbows and knees and gently lower your knees to touch the outside of your elbows.**

2. **Spread your fingers wide for better support. Keeping your elbows bent, form a ledge to rest your knees on.**

3. **Lean your torso forward as you drop your head downward and place some of your body weight onto your elbows.**

4. **Keep pushing gently forward with your toes and try to lift your feet off the floor as you balance your knees on your elbows, as shown in Figure 16-1.**

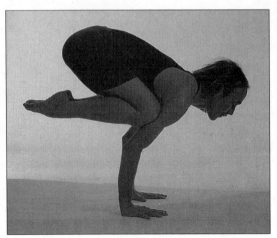

Figure 16-1:
The Crane
builds
balance and
upper-body
muscles.

5. **Hold this position for 5 complete breaths, then lower your feet back to the floor and relax in the Seated Angle Pose (see the Cheat Sheet or Figure 8-1).**

After you succeed in the Crane position, try the Running Man variation.

1. **Follow Steps 1 and 2 for the Crane Pose, then walk both feet over to the outside of your right elbow.**

2. **Drop your head and left shoulder down low to your left side. Place both your knees on top of your right elbow.**

3. **Spread your fingers wide, lean forward and try to lift your feet off the floor as you balance both knees on your right elbow.**

Make sure to keep your right elbow bent to provide support for your knees.

4. **As you find your balance, try to straighten your legs and balance your whole body parallel to the floor, while remaining balanced on your right elbow.**

5. **Balancing on your elbows, split your legs, moving your left leg forward and your right leg back, keeping your feet pointed, supporting all of your weight with your arms and hands (see figure 16-2).**

6. **Hold this position for 5 complete breaths.**

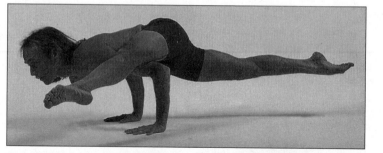

Figure 16-2:
The Running
Man
requires
strength and
balance.

7. **Lower your feet back down to the floor and return to the Downward Facing Dog position.**

8. **Repeat on your left side.**

9. **After doing both sides, relax into the Seated Angle Pose.**

Building more strength with the Flying V Pose

Defying gravity in the Flying V pose, another really good strength building exercise. This beautiful posture takes a combination of abdominal and arm strength and gives back muscle strength and physical confidence.

1. **Begin in the Easy Posture: Sit straight with your legs crossed, then, uncross your legs and bend your knees up toward your chest, placing your feet flat on the floor.**

2. **Place your hands on the floor beside your hips. Lean back on your hands, straighten your arms, and lift your hips and legs straight up into the air, as shown in Figure 16-3.**

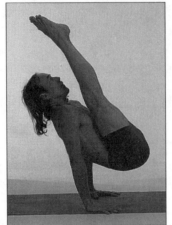

Figure 16-3:
Work slowly
toward
mastering
the Flying V
— you'll be
glad you did.

3. **Hold this position for 5 deep breaths, then lower your legs back down to the floor and relax in the Easy posture again for a few breaths.**

Chapter 17

Riding with Lance Armstrong: Endurance Postures

. . . .

In This Chapter

▶ Building strength and endurance with Power Yoga

▶ Setting the pace of your workout

▶ Boosting endurance through cross-training

▶ Adding oomph to your Power Yoga routine

. . . .

*O*ne of the Power Yoga benefits that folks tend to forget about is its incredible ability to build endurance. Building up a big head of steam through tough, physical exercise is a real show of strength — but sustaining that energy output over a long period of time takes endurance. Regular Power Yoga practice lets you endure a long and powerful workout, and come out smelling like a rose. (Well, maybe you won't smell like a rose, but you won't feel the thorns of fatigue, either.)

Throughout this chapter, I give you tips on how to successfully build endurance through your Power Yoga practice. I show you how to direct the power of your body and your mind to extend your endurance beyond its current limits, and give you some powerful cross-training exercises to do within your endurance training. Last, but not least, I share some Power Yoga tips for building your regular practice routine into a high-endurance marathon. And the great part of this marathon is that you're always the winner!

Working It: Aerobic and Anaerobic Yoga

Power Yoga's linking movements (*vinyasas*) are the important *aerobic* elements that put the *power* in Power Yoga. But don't forget that Power Yoga's pushing, flexing, and balancing postures all work to build strength, too. Strength-building, or *anaerobic*, exercise is another powerful benefit of regular Power Yoga practice. The combination of aerobic and anaerobic exercises in a well-balanced Power Yoga routine builds endurance. Aerobic exercise is any exercise that increases your circulation and works your heart and lungs for more than a few minutes.

After the first 10–15 minutes of your workout, you begin to draw upon your endurance training; the benefits of this training can see you through for hours (see Figure 17-1).

Figure 17-1: The combination of aerobic and anaerobic exercise builds endurance training into your Power Yoga workouts.

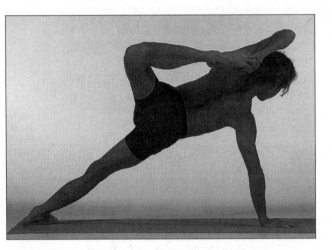

I consistently divide *vinyasas* into three categories — cool, warm, and hot. The categories are based on the amount of physical effort required to work through the *vinyasa;* the hotter the *vinyasa,* the more effort it requires. As a result, a hot *vinyasa* increases your heart rate and creates a semi-aerobic exercise all by itself.

In a well-balanced Power Yoga routine, you begin with a cool *vinyasa* and build toward hotter *vinyasas* as your workout progresses. This gradual build-up of heart rate, respiration, body heat, and energy output works to increase your endurance. In the course of your Power Yoga workout, you strengthen your muscles, work your cardiovascular system, and revitalize your lungs. All of this results in extending your body's endurance.

Pacing Yourself

Notice that in all my references to the process of improving your endurance, I refer to "building" it. That's because you can't increase your endurance overnight. If you run into the Yoga studio, charge through one pose after another, and use the hottest *vinyasas* to connect your routine together, you can expect to come out of the studio with nothing to show for your effort but sore muscles.

Using your body-mind connection

I'm sure you know that the state of your mind plays a big role in the condition of your body and the progress you make in your Power Yoga practice. But when it comes to building your endurance, you'll never find a more powerful tool than your body-mind connection.

When you tell yourself that you can't do something, you're doomed to fail, right? But if you tell yourself that you can and will succeed, you've overcome the biggest hurdle between you and your success. Just make sure that you choose a Power Yoga routine that fits your current ability — one that challenges you, but is not beyond your capacity. No one succeeds in weightlifting if, on his first workout, he tries to bench press 500 pounds.

When you're working to build endurance in your Power Yoga practice, a positive attitude is your best friend. By visualizing your success and keeping a strong vision of your eventual success with you as you move through your routine, you actually feel stronger, more flexible, and more capable of going the distance. This body-mind connection is a big source of your Power Yoga energy; you can channel that energy into anything you choose to accomplish.

After I finish a Power Yoga routine, I can tackle the most incredibly demanding physical work and get it done efficiently. My mind is more organized, and my body works in a stronger and more organized manner, too. Power Yoga helps you do more — and do it better. You can use the benefits of the body-mind connection to help improve your endurance in other sports, recreational activities, or just your daily "survival" routine.

To build endurance, you have to gradually condition your body — internally and externally. Think of your Power Yoga routines as you would think about running up a hill. If you want to be successful, you have to pace yourself and save enough energy to get all the way to the top. After you reach the top, you can easily glide down the other side. Within your Power Yoga routine is an energy summit; you have to pace yourself to make it past the energy summit, so you can glide comfortably through the last part of your workout.

Before you begin a Power Yoga routine, you should have a good idea of what it demands of you, so that you can pace yourself for the best workout experience. Take a look at the elements in your routine, and then figure up the routine's demands in these areas:

- ✔ **Energy:** How much energy will you have to expend?
- ✔ **Strength:** What kind of strength will the postures require?
- ✔ **Flexibility:** How much stretching and bending is involved?
- ✔ **Endurance:** How much endurance will you need to meet these demands?

In other words, take a good, hard look at your routine before you start working through it. Keep the middle and end of your routine in mind as you start — take the time you need to safely and comfortably move through your entire routine. You can increase the intensity and duration of your Power Yoga exercise as you become more comfortable, and slowly build greater endurance. Remember that slow and steady is the best way to build your Power Yoga practice — and your endurance.

For aerobic exercise to be beneficial, you need to create an optimal overload condition — one that won't kill you, but will make you stronger. You need to know that you are exercising at a level that does not overtax your heart but is still intense enough to condition your heart, lungs, and muscles. You can learn how much power is right for you in one of two fairly reliable ways. For both, you need to know your target heart rate, which is 60–75 percent of your maximal heart rate. The Karvonen Formula is used to calculate your maximal heart rate. This formula takes into account your age and your resting heart rate, which tends to be lower when you are fit and not stressed. You need to know your maximal heart rate (your highest possible heart rate) which, unless you want to have it tested in an exercise lab, can be reasonably estimated by subtracting your age from 220. You also need to take a one-minute pulse. Then you can plug these numbers into a simple formula that will let you know your target heart range.

Use these steps to calculate your target heart range:

1. **Subtract your age from 220.**

   This is your estimated maximal heart rate.

2. **Subtract your resting heart rate from your maximal heart rate.**

   This is your heart rate reserve.

3. **Multiply your heart rate reserve by .60.**

4. **Add your resting heart rate to the answer you got in Step 3.**

   This is the lower end of your target heart rate range.

5. **Multiply your heart rate reserve by .75.**

6. **Add your resting heart rate to the answer you got in Step 5.**

   This is the higher end of your target heart rate range.

After you begin your Power Yoga workout and you feel that you're really turning up the heat, take a six-second pulse and add a 0. For example, if your six-second count is 18, your heart rate is 180. If the number you get is higher than your target range, ease up a bit.

If all this seems a bit too, well, technical, you can use an alternative method. It's called the "rate of perceived exertion," a method developed by Gunner Borg.

Traveling companions on the endurance trail

When you start down the road to big-time endurance, don't travel alone. Your Power Yoga practice can build your endurance, but you'll build it faster and take it farther if you partner your practice with some other good fitness pals. To create the most successful endurance program with Power Yoga, you need to get adequate rest and adequate sleep, and eat a healthy diet.

Your Power Yoga practice gives you big benefits, but it takes some big "draws" on your body's resources, too. By combining these good-health habits with your regular Power Yoga training, you'll give your body the extra "oomph" it needs to keep the engine stoked and churning as you build strength, flexibility, and endurance.

Follow the laws of nature in caring for your body:

✔ Combine the proper foods in your diet with plenty of pure water and fresh juices.

✔ Breath slow and deep to feed your body all the fresh air that it needs.

✔ Make sure that you're giving your body ample rest — which means occasionally taking days off from strenuous workouts and always getting a full night of restful sleep.

You can progress steadily and powerfully through your Power Yoga practice if you take care of your body.

The rate of perceived exertion scale lets you assign a number between 6 and 20 to how hard you are working. Numbers between 6 and 10 are in the very, very light to very light range. Numbers over 16 are in the hard to very, very hard range. Numbers between 11 and 15 are where you want to be, because these tend to correspond to the target heart range. Researchers have found that a good relationship exists between how hard you think you're working and the more precise measurements that can be done in a lab.

Exercise scientists think that cross-checking your rate of perceived exertion with your actual target heart range is important; within a few weeks of cross-checking, you should know fairly precisely how hard your heart is working. You make your best gains when you are in the target zone. More is definitely not better for heart health, so don't let your lust for power turn the heat into a destructive fire.

Cross-Training for an Endurance Boost

As with other areas of your Power Yoga practice, you can boost your endurance-building capabilities by combining other activities with Power Yoga in your weekly fitness routine. You might try doing some endurance weight training, for example, where you do a long series of lifts using very light weights. Or try some endurance bicycling that involves some uphill biking — endurance biking builds strength *and* endurance.

You also can intersperse some uphill hiking into your weekly fitness routine to build aerobic endurance and strengthen your legs. And don't forget the benefits of long power walks. Any of these activities, combined with regular Power Yoga practice, will give your endurance training an incredible boost. And cross-training is a great way to increase the other benefits of Power Yoga — from strength training to weight loss and beyond. I give you a sample cross-training table in Chapter 4 — check it out.

Building Endurance in Any Power Yoga Routine

In Chapters 11, 12, and 13, I list Power Yoga routines that offer a balance of aerobic and anaerobic exercises. Any of these routines, or any balanced Power Yoga routine that you create, will deliver endurance-building benefits over time. Continued, regular practice combined with careful attention to your breathing, relaxation, and personal limits is a guaranteed path to better physical endurance. Slowly working your way up from the mildest of these routines to the most strenuous is another way to guarantee that you continually expand your endurance through Power Yoga.

But if you want to boost the endurance-building power of any Power Yoga routine, you can do a bit of "customization." To add an extra endurance factor to any Power Yoga routine, follow these suggestions:

- ✔ Increase your Sun Salutations to twice (or even more) the normal number of repetitions.

- ✔ Slowly add more *vinyasas* until you eventually have a connecting link between every posture.

- ✔ Always keep moving during your routine — save your relaxation time for the end of practice.

The endurance-building benefits of Power Yoga are just some of the many ways that this practice can help you become stronger, healthier, and more active. With regular Power Yoga practice, some cross-training activities, a good diet, and a positive, powerful attitude, you'll have strength and energy to spare; you can take life in stride and keep that big Power Yoga grin on your face through it all.

Chapter 18

Pumping Up Like Arnold for Ripping Abs and Arms

. . . .

In This Chapter

▶ Building better abs, the Power Yoga way

▶ Practicing some postures for strong abs

▶ Strengthening arm and shoulder muscles

▶ Working through a Power Yoga routine for abs and arms

. . . .

Television advertisements for the latest flavor of home exercise equipment always include at least one close-up of someone's rippling (and highly oiled) upper body. Who wouldn't want to have those washboard abs and bulging arm and shoulder muscles? Well, you don't have to haul yet another high-priced home-gym-turned-clothes-rack into your bedroom to get firm, powerful abdominal and arm muscles. Power Yoga offers some of the best workout options you'll find for building upper-body strength.

In this chapter, I show you some great Yoga postures for building abdominal and arm muscles. But first, I recommend that you take a minute to think about your abdominals and what role they play in your daily life, how you can avoid back problems by strengthening your abdominal muscles, and how to use *bandhas* (muscle locks) to give your abs the most effective workout.

I show you how to strengthen your arms through regular Power Yoga practice, and I walk you through an exercise targeted specifically at toning and strengthening arm and shoulder muscles. I also tell you about cross-training to boost your Power Yoga benefits and balance your progress. And, of course, I finish the chapter with a full Power Yoga "abs and arms" routine. The exercises in this chapter are fun, but they offer you some serious challenges, too. So grab your Yoga workout clothes from the ski machine, pull your yoga mat out from behind the multi-flex gym-on-a-rope, and get ready to power up those abs and arms!

Working Those Abs with Power Yoga

I wasn't born a Power Yogi, you know. I practiced softer forms of Yoga for years before Ashtanga and Power Yoga was practiced in America. When I first launched into heavy-duty Power Yoga routines, I couldn't believe how sore my abdominal muscles were after the workout. But over the weeks and months, I also noticed how much my abs had strengthened. Those strong abdominal muscles were an unexpected gift of my regular Power Yoga practice.

If you've ever seen a video of Power Yoga or visited a Power Yoga class, you've probably noticed how much the students work their abs. In fact, the *vinyasas* that connect individual Yoga exercises are powerful abdominal-strengthening tools. Those linking movements are also good for working your arms and back. (If you have any doubts about how a *vinyasa* can improve your abdominal muscles, turn to Chapter 10 and check out the UFO *vinyasa.)*

Beyond the *vinyasas,* though, many Yoga postures involve the specific use of your abdominal muscles and can strengthen these muscle groups quite well. You'll find some of these later in this chapter, of course!

Accumulating strong abs

If you think that tightening your abdominal muscles is all about looking buff on the beach, you're missing some of the more important benefits of toning this muscle group. Sure, toned abs make you look great, but they also can help you prevent back injuries. Strong abdominals also improve your posture — again, making you look better, but at the same time, protecting your back from the strain of supporting your mid-torso weight. So strengthening your abs makes you look better *and* feel better.

When those abdominal muscles are strong and tight, you feel like doing more because your whole body feels stronger all day. Whether you're chasing kids around the yard, rushing through the airport with a laptop and a full brief-case, or just taking a long, quiet walk, the increased strength and back-support you gain from strong abs will help you keep going longer and stronger.

Using bandhas to build abdominal muscle strength

Bandhas, or muscle locks (see the Cheat Sheet), are an extremely effective Power Yoga "helper" for your body. You engage the muscle or energy locks during your Power Yoga postures and *vinyasas* to help strengthen your postures and boost the benefits of your workout.

Back problems and your abdominal muscles

Most people don't associate back problems with weak abdominal muscles. But weak abdominal muscles don't just contribute to back problems; they can actually cause back problems to occur. When your abs are weak, your posture is probably poor, making it easier for the vertebrae to slip out of alignment or for simple movements to result in pulled back muscles. Abdominal muscles help to support and align your spine, hips, and stomach. By strengthening your abdominal muscles through Power Yoga, you actually are strengthening your back muscles at the same time. If you suffer from frequent backaches — especially ones that occur if you're on your feet for any length of time — you should suspect that your abs are contributing to the problem. Strengthen those abs, and see if the backaches let up. (In any case, you'll look better and feel better with those toned and flexible abdominal muscles!)

The two main *bandhas* used in Power Yoga are the *Mula bandha* and *Uddiyana bandha. Mula bandha* is sometimes called the *root lock* because it's located at the base of your spine. *Uddiyana bandha* means "flying up," because when you engage this *bandha,* you actually lift your stomach, which then draws up your diaphragm. Although you typically use these *bandhas* together, the *Uddiyana bandha* in particular works directly to firm your abdominal muscles.

Engaging a *bandha* is similar to clenching your fist. When you clench your fist, the muscles in your arm grow tight and strong. When you engage your *bandhas,* you tighten all your lower abdominal muscles from the inside, which helps tone your internal organs and strengthen your abs.

Cross-training to build abs

I don't believe that any one perfect exercise exists for building your abs — not even Power Yoga. We now know that genetics play a huge role in whether you have those perfect abs, anyway. But for those of us who weren't born with washboards on our midriffs, the best way to build strong, rippling abdominals is to combine some good cross-training exercises with regular Power Yoga practice.

I talk lots in this book about the benefits of cross-training because it's such an important concept. Just as you have to eat a varied, well-balanced diet in order to get the best nutrition, you need to combine a variety of activities to have a good physical training program. To build your abdominal muscle strength, you should consider some basic calisthenics or dance, martial arts training, swimming, or weightlifting. Although Power Yoga is a well-balanced workout program, you gain real benefits by incorporating one or more cross-training activities into your schedule. I make some recommendations for cross-training in Chapter 4.

You can also cross-train by practicing some traditional Yoga postures; good abdominal exercises don't always have to be killers, either. For example, the Upside Down Walker and the Cat Stretch (both described in Chapter 9) are easy exercises, but they still deliver a respectable abdominal workout.

Following the Killer Abs and Arms Routine

Here's my no-fail, best-ever Power Yoga routine for building buff arms, abs, and shoulders. The best way to use this routine is to alternate it with a basic routine from Chapter 11, 12, or 13, whichever of those workouts best suits your present level of practice.

To get the maximum benefit for your arms and abs, you should do a *vinyasa* between each exercise. You can vary these *vinyasas* between hot, warm, and cool versions. If you need a refresher on the *vinyasa* choices, see Chapter 10, where I describe all the versions. Then choose your weapons, and add them to this routine.

Table 18-1	Killer Abs and Arms Routine	
Posture	**Duration**	**Reference**
Cat Stretch	2 repetitions	Figures 9-4 & 9-5
Downward Dog Pushups	10 repetitions	Figure 12-1
UFO *Vinyasa*	1 repetition	Figures 10-5,10-12, 10-3b, 10-13
Energy Saver Salutation	5 repetitions	Figures 10-1–10-6
Feeling Your Oats Salutation	5 repetitions	Figures 10-1a, 10-6–10-8
Monkey Jump	1 repetition	Figures 10-16–10-18
Flying Warrior	5 breaths each side	Figure 13-3
Missing Link	1 repetition	Cheat Sheet
Seated Forward Bend	5 breaths/2 repetitions	Figure 11-4
UFO	1 repetition	Figures 10-13,10-5,10-12, 10-3b, 10-13
Yoga Sit-Ups	5 repetitions	Figure 18-1
UFO	1 repetition	Figures 10-13,10-5,10-12, 10-3b, 10-13
Incline Plane	5 breaths	Figure 12-6

Posture	Duration	Reference
UFO	1 repetition	Figures 10-13,10-5,10-12, 10-3b, 10-13
Cobra	5 breaths	Figure 10-3a
UFO	1 repetition	Figures 10-5,10-12, 10-3b, 10-13
Locust	5 breaths	Figure 13-7
UFO	1 repetition	Figures 10-5,10-12, 10-3b, 10-13
Peacock	5 breaths	Figure 18-2
UFO	1 repetition	Figures 10-5,10-12, 10-3b, 10-13
Boat to Scale	5 breaths/5 repetitions	Figures 11-6; 12-12
UFO	1 repetition	Figures 10-13,10-5,10-12, 10-3b, 10-13
Handstand	5 breaths	Figure 13-9
UFO	1 repetition	Figures 10-13,10-5,10-12, 10-3b, 10-13
Crane	5 breaths/2 repetitions	Figure 16-1
UFO	1 repetition	Figures 10-13,10-5,10-12, 10-3b, 10-13
Bridge	5 breaths/2 repetitions	Figure 13-10
UFO	1 repetition	Figures 10-13,10-5,10-12, 10-3b, 10-13
Yoga breathing	20 breaths	Cheat Sheet
Relaxation	5–15 minutes	Figure 14-1

Pursuing powerful postures for strong abdominal muscles

Almost every aspect of Power Yoga involves the use of your abdominal muscles — sitting straight, standing straight, twisting, bending, stretching, and almost every other movement you make in a Power Yoga routine calls upon your abs. And as you develop your abs, you'll discover that stronger abs make for a better practice. You can keep going longer, have better balance, and maintain better muscle control when your abdominal muscles are strong and toned.

The postures I list in this section are especially good at giving your abs a workout. Try to incorporate them into your regular Power Yoga workout, to direct some special attention on building abdominal strength.

Strengthening your abs with the Scale Pose

The Scale Pose, which I detail in Chapter 12, has you balance your body's weight between your hands as you lift your crossed knees upward. This exercise is great for strengthening your stomach muscles, and it works wonders for your arm and shoulder muscles. If you're interested in building abdominal strength, I recommend that you add this posture to your regular Power Yoga routine.

Firming your abs with Yoga sit-ups

Yoga sit-ups really firm your abdominal muscles. Yoga sit-ups can be very hard or relatively simple, depending on which version you try. I've incorporated a beginner's variation in this exercise.

The more advanced variation of this exercise requires strong abdominal muscles, and it's not for everyone. So don't panic if you can't jump right to the advanced version. Regular practice with the beginner's version of Yoga sit-ups will get your abdominals in good shape so you can tackle the advanced variation (and really firm up your abs).

Start firming your abs by following these steps:

1. **Lie on your back in the Corpse Position (see the Cheat Sheet), with your feet about 12 inches apart and your hands by your sides, palms facing up.**

   Your mind should be calm and relaxed.

2. **On an inhalation, stretch your arms over your head and stretch your legs out long (see Figure 18-1a); completely fill your lungs with air as you stretch.**

3. **On an exhalation, engage your *bandhas*, fold forward at the waist, and lift your hands and feet off the floor, as shown in Figure 18-1b.**

   Ideally, as you lift your torso and legs upward, you will extend your arms in front of you parallel to the floor.

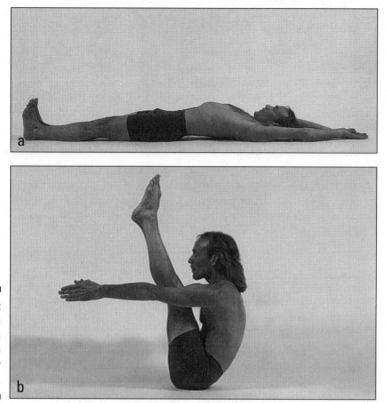

Figure 18-1:
The Yoga sit-up is a great way to firm your abs.

4. **As soon as you reach your maximum sit-up position, inhale, release your *bandhas*, and slowly lie down, with your arms stretched out over your head.**

   Don't worry if you can't even think about doing these sit-ups right now; I have a variation for you. As you start to sit up, lift your arms up as you sit forward and bend your knees. Sit up as far as you can, and then slowly lower your body to the floor.

5. **Repeat the sit-ups 5–10 times.**

6. **On the last repetition, hold your upward position by grasping your legs; hold this position for five slow, deep breaths.**

   If you're doing the beginner's variation, just balance on your hips with your knees bent and your arms parallel to the floor.

7. **Relax into the Corpse Pose for five slow, deep breaths.**

Building Strong Arms and Shoulders

When you do Power Yoga, you're actually doing lots of weightlifting. You push, lift, and pull your body's weight throughout a typical Power Yoga routine. In many (if not most) Yoga exercises, you stretch your arms and shoulders and use them to balance your weight. *Vinyasas* require lots of weightlifting work, too, as you lift your body forward and backward to move from one posture to the next. All this weightlifting spells big gains for your upper-body strength.

And don't forget that in Power Yoga, you're exercising your arms and shoulders with a balanced, yogic approach — stretching, counter-stretching, pushing, pulling, and constantly feeding your cardiovascular and muscular system with an ample flow of strong, oxygenated blood. All in all, a good Power Yoga workout is a great arm- and shoulder-building experience.

Strong arms benefit your Power Yoga practice, too. Not only do they help you build body heat and momentum through strong *vinyasas,* but strong arms also contribute to your stability and balance. Combined with good abdominal strength, those strong arms and shoulders help you take your Power Yoga practice to more powerful levels.

Remembering to cross-train

You've seen how Power Yoga practice gives you good arm and shoulder workouts. And because you use your arm muscles in almost everything you do during an active day, in a way, you're constantly cross-training those muscles. But you still should incorporate some specific cross-training activities into your fitness program, for the maximum "oomph" in your arm and shoulder strength training.

To get a good, well-rounded arm and shoulder workout, try adding some light calisthenics, chin-ups, push-ups, or light weightlifting to your fitness schedule. Swimming, baseball, archery, and football also help strengthen and tone arm and shoulder muscles — at least on one arm unless you're ambidextrous. Combined with regular Power Yoga practice, these activities can give you the good upper-body workout you need.

Balancing the build-up

When you work your arms, you should exercise both the front and back muscles. Most strengthening exercises tighten your arm and shoulder muscles, so don't forget to follow them up with stretching and lengthening postures. Remember that balance is important in every phase of your Power Yoga progress.

You also can maintain a balanced workout by varying the Yoga postures that you include in your Power Yoga routines. Lots of Yoga postures are good for building strong arm and shoulder muscles, and if you tried to do them all in a single workout, you might not survive! So mix things up a bit, and vary the postures and their repetitions from day to day. Variety is the spice of Power Yoga, after all. (Isn't that how that saying goes?)

Strutting and flexing with the Peacock (Mayurasana)

In the spirit of "all things balanced," I want to show you a great exercise for your arms and shoulders that *also* gives you a powerful workout for your abdominal muscles. How's that for a two-fer? This excellent exercise combines the use of your abdominal muscles and arms as you create a beautiful (although difficult) pose that resembles a peacock.

If you're a beginner, don't try to rush into this posture. This is an intermediate to advanced exercise that involves some difficulty. It demands strength and flexibility, especially in the wrists. If you can't do this posture, don't worry. Many other Power Yoga postures will help you build strong arms and shoulders.

1. **Support your body on the floor, with your hands directly under your shoulders and your knees directly under your hips; keep your back straight and parallel to the floor.**

2. **Bend your arms, touching your forehead to the floor.**

3. **Move your hands so that your fingers face your toes and your palms touch the floor; bend your elbows toward your abdominal muscles, trying to place your elbows below your navel and as close to your pubic bone as you can.**

4. **Push with your bent legs to move some of your weight forward toward your shoulders and take some of the tension off your wrists.**

   As you shift your weight forward, you will begin to balance, with your hands, wrists, and forearms supporting more and more of your weight.

5. **Lift your head, and support yourself on your forearms; straighten your legs completely, and rest on your toes and your hands; direct your vision forward.**

6. **Continue shifting your weight forward, and try to lift your feet off the floor as you balance your entire body parallel to the floor (see Figure 18-2).**

   You must tighten your abdominal muscles, and use your back and arm muscles to hold this pose. If you find this too difficult on your wrists, you can turn your hands slightly outward with your fingers pointing to the sides rather than pointing at your toes.

Figure 18-2:
The
Peacock
builds
arm and
shoulder
strength
and it works
abdominal
muscles,
too.

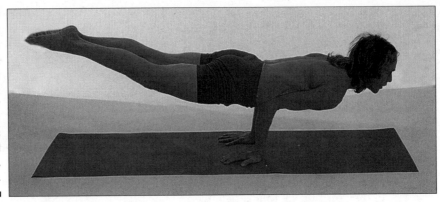

7. **Hold this position for five very slow, deep breaths.**

8. **Lower your legs to the ground, bend your knees, sit back into a kneeling posture, and shake out your wrists a bit to release the tension; exhale, and relax.**

Part V
Enhancing Your Practice

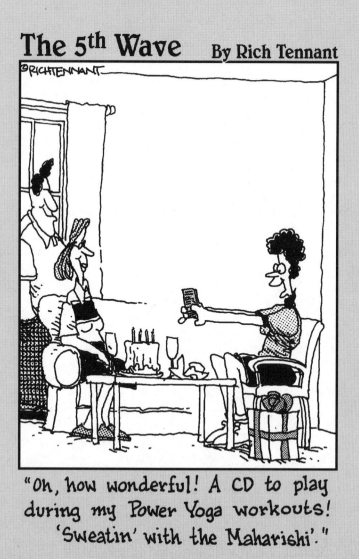

The 5th Wave   By Rich Tennant

"Oh, how wonderful! A CD to play
during my Power Yoga workouts!
'Sweatin' with the Maharishi'."

In this part . . .

A Power Yoga practice can (and of course, I think it
should) last a lifetime. In these chapters, I give you
exercises you can do with while you're pregnant, exercises
you can do with a partner, and exercises you can do in
your active golden years. I also share some tasty recipes
to help keep your Power Yoga body humming along.

Chapter 19

Empowering Women

The old saying, "It's a man's world," sure doesn't apply in the Power Yoga studio. Although Yoga was originally a male-dominated practice, today the tide has turned, and in the West, yoginis outnumber yogis. Women have been drawn to Yoga for some very good reasons. In addition to the fitness workout it delivers, Power Yoga helps women deal with the physical and psychological changes of their hormonal cycles, including menstruation, pregnancy, childbirth, and menopause. And women have discovered the benefits of using Power Yoga to fend off stress while they build strength, endurance, and flexibility.

In this chapter, I tell you how Power Yoga can help you take advantage of all the benefits it offers you as a yogini. After you understand how Power Yoga can help alleviate symptoms of menstruation, you can choose from custom routines and recommended poses for easing cramps and backaches during your monthly cycle. This chapter also gives you information about the benefits of a Power Yoga pregnancy, along with great workout suggestions for when you're practicing for two.

Turning On Your Yoga Power

Life is always shuffling the deck, and as a woman, you never know what cards are coming your way. In addition to the day-to-day stresses of family, finances, career, and that never-ending list of obligations to go somewhere and do something, women get the added wild cards of PMS, pregnancy, menstruation, and menopause. Power Yoga is a woman's trump card for dealing with whatever life throws your way. From *menarche* (your first menstrual cycle) to menopause and beyond, Power Yoga helps you make the most of all the times of your life.

Every teacher has his or her own suggestions for how you should or shouldn't use Yoga at different times in your life. But remember that you're unique, and you have to find your own best way to use Power Yoga in your life. Women are still experimenting with Yoga and its effects on their hormonal changes. Some women, for example, love Downward Facing Dog and find it relaxing and meditative. Others sweat buckets every second they're in the posture and eagerly anticipate its end.

Don't be afraid to carefully explore your body and your Yoga practice. With a quiet mind, you can hear and listen to your body's wisdom and discover what Power Yoga path is right for you.

Herbs that help females

Increasingly, women are seeking herbal remedies for relief from menstrual cramps, nausea during pregnancy, hormonal fluctuations that precede menopause, and so on. If you visit any natural foods store, you can find shelves full of herbal extracts and preparations.

One of the most common problems women suffer in connection with monthly hormonal fluctuations is menstrual cramps. Many women have found old-fashioned ginger to be an effective remedy for these cramps. You can buy some great natural ginger drinks at your health store, brew yourself a cup of ginger tea, or add a few tablespoons of freshly grated ginger to

apple juice. Raspberry leaf is another old-fashioned tea herb that's getting new attention for its ability to help some women overcome nausea during pregnancy. Dong quai, cayenne, sarsaparilla, and blessed thistle are all considered by some to be helpful herbs for women. Herbs can be powerful allies, but you need to use them with care and attention. Be mindful of possible allergies and side effects, and don't take or use anything that doesn't clearly list its ingredients.

For more information on herbs for women, check out *Herbal Remedies For Dummies* by Christopher Hobbs (Hungry Minds, Inc.).

Cycling with Power

Every month, from puberty to menopause, women go through the menstrual cycle. Although menstruation is common to all women, each woman responds to it differently. Some women whip through it without a twinge of pain or discomfort; for others, menstruation can be a painful ordeal. And a woman's menstruation experience can change as she ages; as a teenager, she may have occasional cramps, but few other problems. At 35, the cramps go away, only to be replaced with headaches, bloating, and other symptoms of PMS.

Whether you're trying to smooth slight discomforts or battling full-blown PMS, Power Yoga is a powerful ally. The physical workout helps your body move through its monthly cycle with less discomfort; and the calming, relaxing benefits of regular Power Yoga practice are irreplaceable for avoiding the whiplash of the hormonal roller coaster. Of course, Power Yoga is even more effective at fighting the negative effects of menstruation if you pair it with some good eating habits (I know you want that chocolate, but try to say no) as you approach your cleansing cycle.

When you practice Power Yoga daily (or almost daily), your monthly cycle becomes part of your ongoing process of rejuvenation; as a result, you don't react as strongly to your body's changes each month. You feel less stressed out. Your body is stronger, your mood is balanced, and the hormonal fluctuations seem a little less powerful. Because your practice brings you more in tune with your body, you're mindful of the changes that your body experiences each month, but you don't dread or resent them. Your monthly cycle is a cleansing process in which your body rids itself of what it doesn't need. A big part of your Power Yoga practice is geared toward flushing your body of toxins in a natural, ongoing cleansing process. Your Power Yoga practice helps smooth the ups and downs of your monthly cycle into one calm, continuous process of renewal.

Figure out what works best for you. Many teachers recommend skipping inversions (upside-down poses — see Chapter 12) during at least the first few days of menstruation — because some folks believe that in these poses you're going against the pull of gravity, which may hinder the cleansing or elimination of toxins. But lots of women practice inversions during menstruation without problems. In a recent article in *Yoga Journal,* doctors say that the old rumors about inversions causing endometriosis are untrue.

Often, you may feel exhausted on the first day or so of your period, so you may want to switch from Power Yoga to a more restorative, slower Yoga practice. Experiment with different postures, and do whatever works best for you. But don't skip Yoga completely, because it can be a big help for cramps, backaches, and other effects of fluctuating hormones.

The following sections offer Power Yoga postures and exercises that can be especially helpful for reducing the negative effects of your monthly cycles.

Uncoiling cramped muscles with the Cobra (Bhujangasana)

The Cobra is a great pose for alleviating cramps. It stretches your abdominal muscles, including the muscles of the uterus. These steps can help you act like a mighty Cobra — enjoy!

1. **Lie down on your stomach, with your arms extended by your sides and your palms facing upward.**

   Turn your head to either side, close your eyes, and relax for a few seconds.

2. **Turn your head face down into the floor, resting on your forehead.**

3. **Bend your elbows, and place your hands under your shoulders.**

   Your feet should be pointed behind you, yet relaxed.

4. **On an inhalation, start slowly lifting your shoulders and torso off the floor, one vertebra at a time — like a snake slowly uncoiling.**

   Lift up on an inhalation as high as is comfortable for you.

   If you have limited flexibility, you can rest on your elbows; if you're relatively flexible, lift your torso higher by extending your arms more.

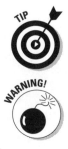

5. **When you reach your maximum comfortable stretch, remain in that position for five deep breaths (refer to Figure 10-3a).**

   If your lower back is stiff and this position causes you pain, separate your legs a bit and allow your ankles to turn outward.

6. **After five deep breaths, exhale and return your torso and shoulders to the floor, take your hands out from under your shoulders, extend your arms back to your sides, turn your head to the side, and relax.**

Take the bite out of cramps with the Upward Facing Dog (Urdhva Mukha Svanasana)

The Sanskrit name for this pose is *Urdhva Mukha Svanasana.* The first two words can be translated as "upward facing." The third word, *Svana,* means "dog." This pose resembles a dog as he stretches out his body after an afternoon nap. I often call this pose Howling at the Moon, and when you try this posture, I think that you'll understand how appropriate the name is.

The Upward Facing Dog is another wonderful abdominal stretch, so it can help you fight off menstrual cramps just like the Cobra. This pose has other benefits as well: It invigorates your spine, opens your chest, and strengthens your arms and shoulders. And if your period leaves you feeling groggy, this pose is the answer — it wakes you up and gives you an energy boost.

Follow these steps to achieve the Upward Facing Dog and check the Cheat Sheet for an illustration:

1. **Lying on your stomach, bend your arms and place your hands under your shoulders, as if you were ready to do a pushup.**

   Rest your chin on the floor, and flex your feet with your toes facing into the ground.

2. **On an inhalation, lift your torso toward the sky, expand your chest, drop your head backward, and look up.**

   During this transition, push with your toes and roll up on top of your feet, with your toes pointed (see Figure 10-2).

3. **Try to support your body on your hands and tops of your feet, with chest expanded, back arched and torso curving upward and your hips slightly off the floor in the Upward Facing Dog Pose (see the Cheat Sheet).**

   Beginners may find this step easier if they place a pillow under their upper thighs.

4. **Hold this position for five complete breaths, and then relax your torso back to the floor.**

Breezing through backaches

The Twist Pose *(ardha matsyendrasana)* is a powerful remedy for backaches. Try this pose the next time you feel the aches and pains of your menstrual period:

1. **Start from the Seated Angle Position (see the Cheat Sheet).**

2. **Bend your left knee, placing your left foot over and on the outside of your extended right leg.**

3. **Lift your arms up, and twist your torso to the left; try to place your right elbow outside your left knee.**

   Place your left hand on the floor behind your back for support (see Figure 19-1).

4. **Look over your left shoulder; hold this position for five complete breaths.**

5. **Untwist your torso to face forward again; straighten both legs in front of you, and come back to the Seated Angle Position.**

   Exhale, and relax.

6. **Repeat this sequence, twisting to the left side this time (place your right leg up over your left leg, and twist your torso to the left).**

7. **After you finish five breaths on each side, return to the Seated Angle Position, sitting with your legs extended in front of you, and relax for a few breaths.**

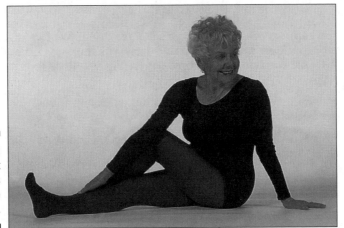

Figure 19-1:
The Twist
helps
relieve
backaches.

Powering Your Way through Pregnancy

There's no better time to hang with Power Yoga than when you're expecting a baby. Power Yoga can do so much to get you through the months of pregnancy and the challenges of childbirth. And the fitness and mental clarity that you build through regular Power Yoga practice can help speed your recovery after childbirth and can help you overcome the stress that new motherhood can bring.

In general, you shouldn't start new activities while you are pregnant, but if you've been practicing Power Yoga all along, keep it up! If not, check with your doctor before you decide to tackle Power Yoga during pregnancy — or find a Power Yoga class that's especially for pregnant women. Whenever you practice Power Yoga, avoid or modify postures that hurt or don't feel comfortable to you (see the section "Modifying postures to create a pregnancy Yoga routine," later in this chapter). And don't forget the power of props (see Chapter 5)! Props provide you with stabilizing support to make your Power Yoga practice more comfortable.

Identifying the best pregnancy poses

Whether you're an experienced yogini or a Power Yoga newcomer, you can benefit greatly from some Yoga postures during pregnancy:

- ✔ Cross-legged seated poses help keep your pelvis open and flexible during birth and continue to work for you even as your baby grows. (Chapter 8 gives you information on seated positions.)

- ✔ All the standing poses of Power Yoga are great for keeping your legs healthy and strong. (Your legs have to carry the extra weight of the baby throughout your pregnancy.) Chapter 10 has many standing poses, too.

- ✔ Yoga breathing exercises provide extra *prana* (life-force energy) and oxygenated blood for you and your baby. See the Cheat Sheet or Chapter 8 for breathing exercises.

Some poses don't feel right when you are pregnant, so you should skip them. For example, lying on your stomach just doesn't work when a baby is growing in there. Some women don't like lying on their backs after a few months of pregnancy, because the weight of the baby blocks their circulation.

Inversions increase circulation in the legs and help stave off varicose veins. However, lots of pregnant women avoid inversions, while others practice them until the baby becomes too large. Some yoginis feel uncomfortable doing back bends during pregnancy, while others find that back bends help ease their aching backs. It's your practice and your pregnancy (not to mention your body), so you need to be cautious and do what works for you.

One big precaution is to avoid extreme stretching. You can still enjoy an active Yoga practice and moderate stretching, but just don't overdo it. Your joints may feel as if they can bend backwards, but that's just your hormones talking — don't listen.

I borrowed the following list from *Yoga For Dummies* by Georg Feuerstein and Larry Payne (Hungry Minds, Inc.). It lists precautions you should take if you're pregnant.

- Avoid extremes, especially deep forward or back bends. Do not strain.

- Avoid sit-ups and postures that put pressure on the uterus.

- Do not jump or move quickly in and out of postures.

- Avoid lying on your stomach.

- Be careful not to overstretch, which you can easily do in pregnancy because of increased hormone levels that cause your joints to become limber.

- Always do a little less than you're used to doing and never hold your breath.

The one thing that is true for everyone is that your Yoga practice changes with your pregnancy. Your baby grows and gets in the way in many of the poses you practice, so you can't go as deep in them. As you progress in your pregnancy, your lungs start getting squished by the baby, so breathing is harder. Practicing Yoga breathing helps, but you probably won't be able to exercise quite as hard as you used to. The baby takes much of your body's energy, too, so you may have the energy only for a mellow practice. All of Power Yoga is good, so don't feel that you are missing out. No matter how much or how little you practice, you'll be blessed with the power of Yoga to get you through the birth.

Cat Tilt and Dog Tilt for a healthy back

Some of the most important things you can do during pregnancy are to stretch your back and your hips. Your back takes on lots of extra work by carrying the weight of the baby, and overworked muscles can end up causing you lots of pain. Power Yoga's gentle twists help keep your back strong and flexible, and its spine-lengthening exercises help create more space for the baby.

When you're carrying a baby, your lower back is prone to strain and tension. Try this Cat and Dog Tilt to keep your lower back happy — especially as the baby gets bigger!

1. **Get on your hands and knees, with your hands directly under your shoulders and your knees under your hips.**

2. **As you inhale, lift your pelvis and tailbone toward the sky, let your back sway downward, and tilt your head upward as you gaze up at the sky.**

   This is the Dog Tilt.

3. **As you exhale, lower your head and hips; tuck your chin into your chest and your tailbone under.**

4. **Arch your back as you try to lift your belly button up toward your spine.**

   This is the Cat Tilt.

5. **Repeat Steps 2 through 4, moving back and forth between the Cat Tilt and the Dog Tilt.**

   Practice your slow, deep Yoga breathing.

Opening your hips with the Butterfly Pose

Ah, the hips! Can there be any better gift than having flexible hips as your baby is being born? Stretch them like crazy as you progress in your pregnancy. Try poses like Expanded Seated Angle (the same as Seated Angle with your legs spread wide, squats (lots of squats!), and the Butterfly Pose.

The Butterfly *(Baddha Konasana)* is a wonderful pose for opening the hips, stretching the muscles of the thighs, and building flexible ankles. The posture also helps increase the blood supply to your abdomen and pelvis.

Follow these steps to achieve the Butterfly:

1. **Sit on the floor in Seated Angle Pose (see the Cheat Sheet).**

2. **Bend your knees, bringing your feet toward the base of your torso, with knees out to your sides and the soles of your feet facing each other.**

3. **Try to bring the soles of your feet together, as you interlock fingers around both feet, and let gravity pull your thighs toward the floor.**

   Maintain good posture as you complete this step.

4. **Lean forward, and try to bring your abdomen out over your feet (refer to Figure 8-7).**

5. **Hold this position for 5–10 complete breaths, and then relax into the Seated Angle Pose.**

Moving your Butterfly up the wall

The Butterfly on the Wall Pose offers the same benefits as the regular Butterfly Pose, but you practice it lying down. This pose lets you take a load off your feet, which is a real tension-releasing bonus when you've been carrying the baby around all day.

1. **Sit on the floor next to a wall and rotate onto your back so you're lying on your back with your buttocks pressed against the wall, your knees bent, and your feet flat against the wall, hip-width apart and about two feet up from the floor.**

2. **Pivot your feet on the wall, turning your heels inward and toes outward, placing your hands on your knees and your elbows on the floor.**

   Lie comfortably in this position, and direct your gaze upward.

3. **Start slow, deep breathing as you pull gently downward and outward on your knees.**

   Hold this position for 10 slow, deep breaths (see Figure 19-2).

4. **Bring the soles of your feet together, but continue resting your feet against the wall, gently pulling downward on your knees with your hands.**

   Hold this position for 5–10 breaths.

5. **Straighten your legs, and extend them up the wall; place your feet about two feet apart and relax for another five slow, deep breaths.**

6. **Bend your knees, lower your legs toward your torso, roll to one side, and slowly return to a sitting position.**

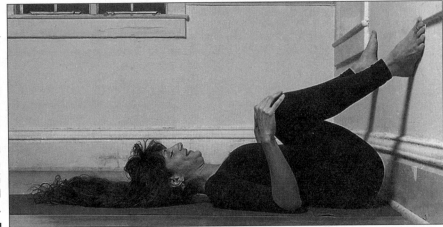

Figure 19-2:
You control the amount of stretch by placing pressure on your knees in the Butterfly on the Wall pose.

Modifying postures to create a pregnancy Yoga routine

You'll quickly determine which Yoga postures do and don't work for you during your pregnancy, and you're sure to change your Power Yoga routine as your body changes over time. But you can modify Power Yoga postures (discussed elsewhere in this book) to build a routine that fits your pregnancy, and that's what this section is about.

To modify Sun Salutations (see Chapter 10):

✔ Place your hands on your hips for support in standing, back-bending exercises.

✔ When you do forward-bending movements from a standing position, separate your feet by 24–36 inches.

✔ As you step one leg back, place your hands on your thigh, pushing down on your thigh as you arch your torso, head, and shoulders upward and drop your head back. This is called the Crescent Moon Pose (see Figure 19-3).

✔ Do the same with your opposite leg forward, and skip the Cobra on the floor.

Figure 19-3:
The Crescent Moon pose stretches the muscles of your stomach, back, and thighs as it lengthens your spine.

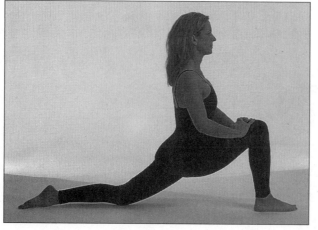

To modify headstands:

- ✔ Unless you're very experienced at the Headstand, practice only the framework or the Half Headstand (refer to Figure 13-11).

- ✔ Form a good base for your headstands with your forearms, and continue as if you are going up into your headstand, but lift one leg up half way. Now try the same thing on the opposite leg. Then come down and relax.

- ✔ As an alternative, lie down on a slant board for a few minutes everyday.

To modify shoulder stands:

- ✔ Use the wall for support to practice your Shoulder Stands. Start from the Butterfly on the Wall position (refer to Figure 19-2). Push your feet against the wall (with your knees bent), and lift your hips. With your bent elbows firmly against the floor and as far underneath your body as you can get them, place your hands on your lower back, lifting into the Shoulder Stand on the Wall (see Figure 19-4).

- ✔ From your Shoulder Stand on the Wall, you can try another variation of the pose by pulling one leg off the wall and down toward your head; hold for a few breaths, and then put that leg back up on the wall and pull the other leg down.

- ✔ When you're finished with your Shoulder Stand, bend your knees, take your hands out from behind your back, and lie back down on the floor. Roll over to one side, and slowly sit up.

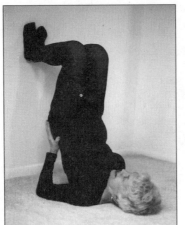

Figure 19-4:
The Shoulder Stand on the Wall gives your legs and feet a break while you exercise.

Keep your legs split in Seated Forward Bends, practice moderate modified spinal twisting, and lots of cat stretching, standing *asanas,* and breathing exercises. Incorporate good nutrition, talk long walks, and get plenty of rest.

Birthing and beyond

Power Yoga practice well prepares you for the major physical challenge of childbirth, by teaching you to use your power tools of Yoga breathing and concentration. Your breathing and concentration can make the hard work of childbirth less difficult and painful.

I've talked to many women who have found Yoga breathing (see the Cheat Sheet) very helpful during labor. It slows you down and helps you to relax. Short, shallow breathing gets the adrenaline pumping in your body and makes you more tense. So when it comes time to give birth, breathe deep, kick back like you're going into the Corpse Pose (see the Cheat Sheet again), and get ready to push that baby out.

And speaking of the Corpse Pose, when you get to the point that it isn't comfortable to lie on your back in the pose, lie on your side with your top leg supported by a blanket and a big pillow. Try a body pillow that is the length of your body. A body pillow makes a nice companion in bed, as well as in your Power Yoga postures.

The birth is only the beginning of your hard work. Over the days and weeks that follow, you're tending to the baby constantly, sleep-deprived, and under lots of stress. Thank goodness for Power Yoga.

Yoga-Hypno-Birthing

Yoga-Hypno-Birthing is a birthing technique growing in popularity. Basically, you practice three important Yoga techniques: sense withdrawal, meditation, and deep relaxation. Some call this self-hypnosis because you are trying to take yourself into a deeply relaxed state. With practice, many women have found that they can relax through anything — even the worst labor pains. You can use the Corpse Pose as a starting point. Many women like to use visualization to think of relaxation as a golden liquid filling their bodies. Try visualization the next time you're in an intense pose, and see whether it may work for you on the big day. For more information on deep relaxation techniques, see Chapter 14.

As soon as your doctor okays it, you can start doing a little Yoga, even if you're only doing breathing exercises in the beginning. A few minutes of Yoga quiet time helps lower your stress level almost as much as a good night's sleep. You should be able to do some simple shoulder stretches (see Chapter 9) and maybe some twists (refer to Figure 19-1) soon after giving birth. You'll be doing lots of lifting and carrying and, if you're nursing, your shoulders are likely to be rounded and get sore. So keep stretching. Be gentle with yourself, and gradually build your practice back to what it once was.

Because you practiced Yoga throughout your pregnancy, your body will more quickly return to its original form. Your practice probably kept your body in tone even as you added the baby's weight; continuing your practice after the birth helps you take the weight back off. And most importantly, Power Yoga helps you keep your head straight and that whole weight thing in perspective by teaching you self-acceptance, patience, and love.

Aging with Power — Menopause

Power Yoga is also a powerful ally for easing the transition from childbearing years into the age of wisdom — menopause. With menopause and the years of hormonal change that precede it come a spectrum of changes. Your body gradually changes as it ages, your ideas and attitudes mature, and your hormone levels go through another series of radical shifts. Power Yoga helps you to deal with these changes without stress.

Not only does Yoga show you how to accept and love your body as it matures, but continued Power Yoga practice keeps your body feeling young and healthy. It helps to level out the hormonal roller coaster, so that you're less likely to experience some of the problematic symptoms like mood swings and hot flashes. Power Yoga also combats moodiness by keeping your mind calm and clear.

Post-menopausal women are at greater risk for some diseases like osteoporosis and heart disease. Power Yoga has many benefits that directly lower the risk of these diseases. Because bones are strengthened through weight-bearing exercise, you can strengthen all the bones of your body. Power Yoga improves the amount of oxygen carried by the blood cells, which reduces the work that the heart has to do. And the aerobic component of Power Yoga strengthens your heart and improves your cardiovascular health. Last but not least, Power Yoga is a stress reducer, and stress is a factor in many diseases, including heart disease. So if you're practicing Power Yoga and eating well, you have a head up on that one. Power Yoga helps keep your muscles and, most importantly, your spine strong, healthy, and flexible. Practicing

Power Yoga is one of the best ways to keep your spine healthy, long, and flexible — so you avoid that stooped-over look so common in many older people.

Recent studies have suggested that weight training helps to prevent osteoporosis, but you get all the benefits of weight-training exercises and more with Power Yoga. Your practice helps give your body the strength-training benefits of weight training, along with the other stretching and circulatory benefits of Power Yoga.

Every day that you practice, you are improving. Whether you're 16 or 60, Power Yoga is one of your biggest allies in getting the most out of your life as a strong, powerful woman. Power Yoga is forever — so keep on keeping strong with Power Yoga!

Chapter 20

Staying Young: Power Yoga for Seniors

In This Chapter

▶ Making Power Yoga work for you

▶ Checking out Power Yoga postures that have seniority

▶ Moving through your own Power Yoga routine

*R*etirement has so many benefits — including extra time to travel, to work in the garden, to visit with family and friends, to go rock climbing, to go parasailing, or finally to surf that big Banzai Pipeline wave in Hawaii. People today don't think of the golden years as a time to kick back and let the world go by. After the kids are out of the house and the career climb is over, you can get out and really enjoy life, however you choose to do it. But if you're out of shape, tired, stiff, and unable to go and do as you please, you can't have much fun — no matter what your age.

That's why Power Yoga becomes your best friend as you hit the post-50 years. At any age, a moderate, regular Power Yoga practice can help you maintain good physical and mental health. But as you reach middle age and beyond, the Power Yoga benefits of increased strength, flexibility, and balance become even more critical. Power Yoga doesn't stop there, either, in helping you stay young as the years roll by. The strong cardiovascular workout of a good Power Yoga practice keeps your heart healthy and helps keep your blood pumping through strong, clean arteries. You'll be more alert and more comfortable in body and mind.

In this chapter, I show you how you can adapt Power Yoga routines to cater to your changing body, lifestyle, and fitness needs. At the same time, I point out a few special considerations to ensure a safe and comfortable Power Yoga journey. The key to any good fitness plan is moderation; with this in mind, I wrap up this chapter with a wonderful Power Yoga routine that should give you just the right amount of heat and power to benefit your mental and physical condition. So put down your gardening tools (or surfboard) for a while, and join me in a look at Power Yoga — the wonder years!

Embracing Power Yoga for All Ages

Beyond death and taxes, you can count on one other thing in life — change. Time passes, and we all get older (and that's the good scenario). But getting older doesn't mean that you have to be less active. In fact, after you jump that 50-year hurdle, a strong, active schedule of physical activity becomes more important than ever.

You don't need to be a mountain climber-in-training to require a good work-out program in your later years; whether you plan to putter around the house or run marathons post-retirement, you need to work at maintaining good fit-ness, strength, and flexibility. Of all the forms of exercise practiced today, Yoga has been proven to be one of the most beneficial exercises for your whole body and mind. Power Yoga has all the benefits of traditional soft-form Yoga, with additional aerobic and muscle-strengthening aspects built in.

Of course, your body does change as it ages, and any fitness routine that you adopt needs to be designed to fit your body's current condition. No single "condition" describes every post-50 body. Countless people in their 60s, 70s, 80s, and even 90s are out climbing mountains and living an active life; other folks are learning to develop a fitness routine late in life, so their bodies need more foundation fitness building. Whatever your condition, the key to build-ing good physical and mental health is to adopt a moderately active program that gets you "up and at it" regularly.

Power Yoga is such a diverse practice. Many Power Yoga exercises are appro-priate for anyone of any age — and most of them have beginner's variations or can be modified to suit older students. If you aren't very active, you can use a beginning-level Power Yoga routine and modify it as necessary to fit your abilities. The key is to practice for short periods on a regular basis; that way, you'll make good progress and build your endurance, strength, and flexi-bility over time.

Understanding Power Yoga benefits for seniors

Seniors get many benefits — reduced prices at restaurants and hotels, and (usually) a prime seat on a crowded bus! But Power Yoga brings you better benefits — the benefits of mental and physical health. If you've been active all your life, you may not notice some of the typical changes of an aging body: Tendons grow shorter, reaction times slow, and breathing can become shal-lower, limiting endurance. Power Yoga fights many signs of aging by offering these benefits:

- ✔ **Increased flexibility:** Power Yoga stretches tendons and muscles to increase flexibility and reduce stiffness.

- ✔ **Strong respiratory and cardiovascular systems:** Regular practice strengthens your respiratory system; as you consume more oxygen during your workouts and Yoga breathing exercises, your lung capacity goes up and your *prana* energy (vital life force) flourishes. By oxygenating your blood, you nourish your entire body — blood, muscles, and brain. You feel refreshed and can think more clearly.

- ✔ **Increased muscle strength:** Recent reports tout the benefits of weightlifting for the elderly, including the prevention of osteoporosis. Power Yoga is a form of weightlifting. Your practice challenges you to lift, push, and pull the weight of your body as you move into one Yoga posture after another.

- ✔ **Better endurance, balance, and coordination:** You grow stronger and build endurance to keep going longer. Power Yoga increases your coordination and balance, too. These are critical factors for leading an active, healthy life and avoiding painful, crippling falls and accidents.

- ✔ **Confidence and peace of mind:** With an energetic, strong, well-balanced and vital body, you feel confident and at peace. You can think of Power Yoga as your ticket to a powerful and happy life throughout the years ahead.

Making Power Yoga work for you

If you think of Power Yoga as a full-throttle, no-holds-barred workout process, you may think that you're not interested in — or not capable of — doing it. Well, if Power Yoga is a wild beast, it's one you're perfectly capable of taming. Just as walking is the beginning phase of running, which is just another step down from marathon racing, Power Yoga can be as gentle or as demanding as you want it to be.

You may have told your kids at one point "you have to crawl before you can walk." The same holds true for your progress toward becoming a Power Yoga student. Don't let fear of your limitations keep you from trying some Power Yoga exercises. After you work through some appropriate Yoga postures, you'll find that you're ready to build a Power Yoga routine that works for you. The more you practice, the more involved and challenging your routine may become. You're in control, so do with Power Yoga as you will.

Considering some cautions

Most people (at any age) aren't in peak physical condition. If you've reached middle age or beyond and you're just beginning to think about getting in shape, you have a tougher road ahead than does someone who's been working out and watching their diet forever. But so what? Lots of people start working out when they're 60, 70, or 80 — it's always a good idea, no matter what your age. But you have to keep the following realities of aging in mind as you build a safe practice program:

- ✔ **Take your time.** As you age, your bones become more brittle even as your joints and muscles become less flexible. With that in mind, be careful when you move in and out of poses. Slow your breathing, and move gently into and out of each Yoga pose.

- ✔ **Use some props.** You're building balance as a Power Yoga student, but initially, your balance may be a bit off. To make sure that you can remain stable and secure during your Yoga postures, use props during your Power Yoga workouts. (I talk about props and their use in Chapter 5.) Props help you build strength and stability faster than if you try to wobble through without them; you'll also enjoy your Power Yoga workouts more.

- ✔ **Grab a partner.** Practicing Power Yoga with a partner is fun! And having a partner to help you balance in some positions, hand you props, or just lend general moral support can make a big difference in your confidence — and safety. A partner is also great to have around if you're going to practice challenging balance postures, especially the upside down postures like headstands and handstands. For complete information on partnering in Power Yoga, see Chapter 22.

- ✔ **Balance your workouts with rest.** Your muscles may not recuperate from a brand new workout as quickly as they did when you were younger. So use a low-level workout routine in the beginning, and if your muscles get sore, back off and rest between workouts. If you get sore and tired every time you do Power Yoga, you'll soon be discouraged by the whole process. If you feel yourself getting sore, take it easier.

Before you launch into becoming a student of Power Yoga, see your doctor for a general checkup. Tell your doctor that you're thinking of doing some Power Yoga exercise, and ask if that is okay, given your present condition. (Take along this book, if you like, so your doctor can see exactly what kind of exercise you're talking about.) Your doctor or health clinic may even be able to recommend some good Yoga programs in your area.

Many Yoga studios ask all their students to bring in a doctor's permission for joining practice sessions. If you take medication of any kind, you should let your Yoga instructor know.

Mixing it up

You may have heard about cross-training for Olympians — well, it applies to you, too! You are never too old to benefit from cross-training. Whether you're 8 or 80, you need to think of cross-training just like those Olympic athletes do — if you want the best, most productive results from your Power Yoga practice. Try walking, bicycling, light weightlifting, or any other type of physical activity that you enjoy.

You'll progress farther in your Power Yoga practice, and you'll be fitter faster. And don't get stuck in a rut with your Power Yoga routines, either. Vary the exercises that you include in your routines, keep trying new and different variations on poses, add repetitions — whatever it takes to keep your practice fun, productive, and progressing. Cross-training is covered in depth in Chapter 4.

Powering Up with a Post-50 Routine

The best way to make a productive start on your way to becoming a post-50 Power Yoga practitioner is to work with a beginning-level routine. The routine in Table 20-1 is a great way to move into Power Yoga. (You can find other suggested beginner postures and routines in Chapter 11.)

If you find that this routine is too difficult using the postures as described in the referenced chapters, don't hesitate to use props (see Chapter 5). And you don't need to work through the entire routine right off the bat. You can try practicing a half or a third of the routine, cutting down the number of recommended repetitions, and so on. In other words, make the workout work for you.

Just remember to do at least a 15-minute relaxation (and here, more is better) wherever and whenever you end!

Table 20-1	Post-50 Power Routine	
Posture	*Duration*	*Reference*
Persuading Posture	5 breaths	Figure 8-3
Upside-Down Walking	5 repetitions	Figure 9-2
Cat Stretch	2 repetitions	Figures 9-4 & 9-5
Seated Forward Bend	2 repetitions	Figure 11-4
Cobra	5 breaths/2 repetitions	Figure 10-3a
Bridge	5 breaths	Figure 13-10

(continued)

Table 20-1 *(continued)*

Posture	Duration	Reference
Spine Toner	5 breaths	Figure 9-1
Missing Link Upward	1 repetition	Figures 10-13–10-16
Extended Side Angle	5 breaths	Figure 13-2
Missing Link Downward	1 repetition	Figures 10-16–10-13
Shoulder Stand	5– 20 breaths	Figure 12-10 b & c
Yoga breathing	5 breaths	Cheat Sheet
Deep relaxation	15–30 minutes	Figure 14-1

Getting Acquainted with Power Yoga Poses for Seniors

After your doctor gives you the green light to begin Power Yoga exercises, you need to find a Yoga class with which you feel comfortable. Ask your friends, look in the telephone book, check with your local Senior Citizens action center, or ask at some local fitness centers. (Check out Chapter 6 and Appendix B to find detailed info on locating and choosing a Yoga center.) When you find a program that looks good to you, talk with the instructor to make sure that the class can accommodate your needs. Then try out a few sample classes to see if everything feels like a good "fit."

No matter what your fitness level is, you should begin your Power Yoga work with some simple postures. Power Yoga makes demands on your body for which other types of exercises may not have prepared you. If you launch your practice by trying to put your feet behind your head while standing upside down on one hand, you're unlikely to enjoy the experience. You are likely to end up shouting for someone to call 911 so the fire department can bring the jaws of life to get you untangled! Take it slow, and work gradually toward building more complex postures into your beginning routines.

Power Yoga isn't a competitive sport. You're in it for you, and you determine what you want to do (or not do) with your practice. Follow your instincts and enjoy the process without feeling out of place, incapable, or silly. Life is an adventure, and developing a regular Power Yoga practice can be one of the most exciting and rewarding trips. Relax, explore, and enjoy.

The following sections describe some Power Yoga exercises that any beginner can enjoy. Check them out for a taste of power.

Developing shoulder relief and leg strength

Try the following gentle Power Yoga exercise routine working from a chair, and see how energized you feel. This exercise helps relieve stress and tension in your shoulders, it expands your chest, and it helps to loosen up tight joints as it strengthens your arms and Legs.

You need two sturdy, straight-back chairs for the last part of this exercise. Place the chairs facing each other, and sit in one. Follow these steps to achieve the Two Chair Stretch and release tension:

Shoulder relief and leg strength with Chair Yoga

1. **Sit in one chair, with your spine straight and shoulders back, hands folded in your lap (see Figure 20-1a).**

   Take a few slow, deep breaths, and relax.

2. **As you inhale, lift your arms out to your sides and over your head with palms touching, as if you are clapping your hands (see Figure 20-1b).**

3. **Exhale, and lower your arms to the starting position (hands in your lap).**

   Keep your shoulders away from your ears as you do this.

4. **Repeat Steps 2 and 3 five times.**

   Remember to inhale as you lift your arms and expand your chest. Exhale as you lower your arms and relax.

5. **Repeat Step 2, inhaling and lifting your arms over your head; exhale as you put weight on your feet and come to a full standing position, with your arms by your sides (see Figure 20-1c).**

6. **Sit back down in your chair, with your spine straight and shoulders back.**

7. **Repeat Step 5 of the exercise for five repetitions.**

   Close your eyes and relax for 10 slow, deep breaths.

8. **Bend forward at the hips, resting your torso on your thighs, and place your arms on the chair in front of you (see Figure 20-1d).**

9. **Hold this position for five slow, deep breaths.**

   You're doing the Two Chair Stretch, which stretches your torso.

10. **Come back to a sitting position and relax.**

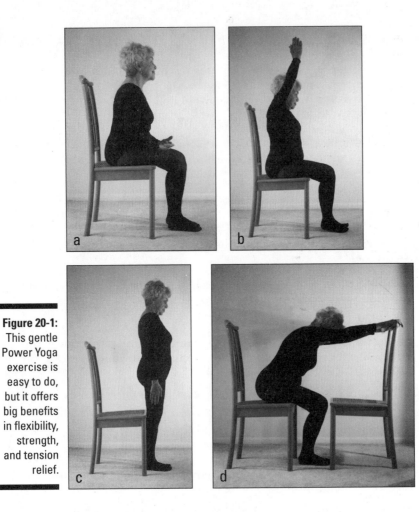

Figure 20-1:
This gentle Power Yoga exercise is easy to do, but it offers big benefits in flexibility, strength, and tension relief.

Propping up your Extended Side Angle Pose

This section provides an easy adaptation of a traditional Power Yoga posture. The traditional Extended Side Angle Pose (discussed in Chapter 13; refer to Figure 13-2) requires you to lunge deep on your right leg with your left leg extended behind you and, at the same time, rest your right hand on the floor. That's some pretty tricky stuff! If you're getting up there in years or you aren't in the greatest physical condition, you can do the same posture without lunging so deeply and with the benefit of some added support. The following version of the Extended Side Angle Pose strengthens legs and tones ankles, knees, and thighs. Using a chair as a prop makes this pose much easier to do, but it doesn't detract from the posture's ability to develop your chest and reduce fat around your waist and abdomen. Opening all the muscles of the rib cage also enhances your ability to breathe.

Have a sturdy chair ready to help you achieve the modified Extended Side Angle Pose:

1. **Start from the Extended Mountain Pose (see the Cheat Sheet)**

   Stand strong and firm with correct posture.

2. **Turn your right foot outward 90 degrees, and turn your left foot in at a 45-degree angle.**

3. **Inhale, lifting your arms to your sides and parallel to the floor.**

4. **Exhale as you lunge, bending your right knee so that your thigh and shin form a 90-degree angle.**

   Your right knee comes directly over your right heel, bringing your thigh parallel to the floor.

5. **Place your right forearm on the seat of the chair for support (see Figure 20-2).**

   Use your right hand to slide into position onto the chair close to your right knee.

6. **Form a 45-degree angle with your body, from your extended left leg (which is back behind you), through your torso, and all the way out to your fingertips.**

   Your left arm is extended up at a 45-degree angle on the same plane as your leg and your torso; your palm should be open, and your hand facing downward.

7. **Turn your head upward, looking up under your arm and toward the ceiling; hold this position for five slow, deep breaths.**

Figure 20-2:
A chair makes the Extended Side Angle Pose a bit easier to do, but it doesn't eliminate its stretching and strengthening benefits.

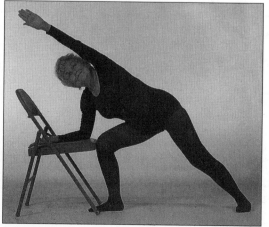

Using wall support for super Shoulder Stands

The Shoulder Stand (see Chapter 12) helps to create harmony and happiness throughout your entire body. In this inverted *asana,* your heart and brain receive a healthy rush of blood; the pose stimulates your endocrine system and gives your thyroid and parathyroid glands a tune up. The Shoulder Stand can even help reverse the effects of varicose veins! Best of all, when you come out of the Shoulder Stand, you feel refreshed and rejuvenated.

You don't have to be a high-wire artist to pull off the Shoulder Stand. The version I show you in this section puts you up against the wall for a perfectly supported and stable experience. By putting your legs up against the wall, you feel more comfortable and less wobbly in this pose.

When you do this exercise, you should have a thick towel or blanket so you can use it to elevate your shoulders and protect your neck from too much tension. Move slowly and carefully, and ask someone to help stabilize your legs when they're in the air in this exercise.

1. **Position yourself near a wall, placing a folded blanket on the floor parallel to the wall.**

2. **Lie down in the Corpse Position (see the Cheat Sheet), with your shoulders on the blanket.**

   Keep your shoulders elevated and your head resting off the blanket. Lie on your back, arms extended by your sides, your feet about one foot apart. Make sure that your palms face upward and your mind is calm and relaxed. Bend your knees, and let your toes touch the wall.

   You don't want to use the blanket as a pillow — because it causes more harm than good. The object is to lift your shoulders and create less tension on your neck.

   Place your body so you have about two inches of blanket beyond the tops of your shoulders. Your body should roll back slightly as you lift up into this posture. When you are completely lifted up into the posture, your shoulders should still be entirely on the blanket, your neck should be free, and your head should be on the floor. Having your neck free means that you can slip your fingers underneath your neck — if you aren't using them to help you hold yourself upside down. The pose should feel comfortable. In fact, you may be surprised at how comfortable it does feel. If you feel a lot of pressure behind your eyes or in your head or if you feel pain in your neck or back, come on down and talk to your friendly Yoga professional to see if this pose can be right for you.

3. **Exhale completely; on an inhalation, place your feet flat on the wall a couple feet above the floor.**

4. **Push your weight into your feet as you lift your hips, supporting your hips with your hands.**

   Tuck in your elbows behind your back, and use your elbows and hands to support your lower back.

5. **Push up into a full wall-supported Shoulder Stand.**

   Hold this position for 5–20 complete breaths (refer to Figure 12-10c).

6. **Inhale again, place your hands under your hips, and push down to lift your hips off the floor.**

7. **Tuck in your elbows behind your back, and use your elbows and hands to support your elevated legs and hips.**

   Ask your helper to steady you so you don't topple to the side.

8. **Extend your legs and torso as high as you comfortably can, remembering to support your back with your hands.**

9. **Hold this posture for 5–20 slow, deep breaths.**

10. **Come down slowly and relax on your back.**

If you have, or may have, osteoporosis, take care doing this pose. It's important not to put weight on your neck vertebrae.

Chapter 21

Practicing Yoga Adjustments and Working with a Partner

. . . .

In This Chapter

▶ Getting the most from Yoga adjustments

▶ Having twice the fun with partner Yoga

. . . .

Years ago, when I first started teaching Yoga, I didn't give my students any hands-on assistance with their Yoga postures. I'd stand at the front of the studio, demonstrate the postures, and give my students plenty of verbal coaching and assistance. Then one day, a woman in the back of the class had trouble hearing my instructions. I walked back to her to explain, and while I was there, I helped her position her arms and legs in the correct pose. As a final touch-up, I gently corrected her posture and spinal alignment. She thanked me and said, "I never could have got this alignment on my own." Years have passed since that day when I learned the value of hands-on assistance in teaching Yoga postures, and today, the practice even has its own name — *Yoga adjustment.*

Don't get me wrong — you certainly can practice Yoga on your own and have a successful practice without the assistance of an instructor or willing friend. But when you're practicing Yoga postures, the hands-on assistance of a Yoga teacher or someone with Yoga experience can be a big help. You'll progress quicker, enjoy postures you aren't able to achieve on your own, and maintain better postures and proper alignment within each pose. Partner work in Yoga is often similar to a Yoga adjustment, but much of the joy of partner work is the fun of sharing the Power Yoga experience.

In this chapter, I discuss how, when, and why you may want to seek out an instructor for Yoga adjustment. I talk to you about the creativity and fun of Power Yoga with a partner. I also show you some effective partner exercises, and how you can turn partner work into an effective Yoga adjustment experience. So what are you waiting for? Grab your partner and get ready to discover the joys of Power Yoga for two.

Using Yoga Posture Adjustments

To get the most from any Power Yoga posture, you must properly align and position every part of your body. Teachers and experienced Yoga students use Yoga adjustments to help others move into and hold each pose properly. Other adjustments modify standard postures to give them added "oomph." Yoga adjustments are helpful and appropriate for students at every level of practice.

You don't have to be a long-term yogi or yogini to offer someone help in achieving a Yoga posture, but you do need to be familiar with the posture that person is attempting. You also can read the steps in Parts III and IV and look at the pictures that describe and illustrate the postures I've supplied, and then use that information to help a fellow student get with the program.

You have to be careful when you're physically moving someone's body position — especially when that person may be balancing or twisting in a precarious pose. Follow these few rules for giving Yoga adjustments:

- ✔ Never give a Yoga adjustment to someone without her permission.
- ✔ Don't attempt to adjust someone in a Yoga posture with which you aren't very familiar.
- ✔ Never adjust against deep resistance. *No forcing.*
- ✔ Don't force your partner's or anyone's knees to the floor.
- ✔ Never adjust directly at a joint.

The bottom line is this: Only the person receiving the adjustment knows exactly how it feels, so you have to communicate with the person you're working with. Make sure that the person knows exactly why you're moving any part of his or her body; also, be sure to explain clearly the final goal for the adjustment you're making. For example, you can say "Your arm needs to be straight and pointing toward the ceiling; I'm just going to straighten your elbow and lift your arm a few inches."

Always have a backup plan, such as a less-dramatic adjustment or a prop to assist with the Yoga posture. And always be gentle when advancing someone into a stretch; it's much better to be too gentle with your adjustment than to injure someone by forcing him into a posture that his body simply isn't ready for. And you also need to be certain that you don't hurt yourself when trying to help a fellow Yoga student achieve a posture. I learned that lesson the hard way. Don't try to take on more weight than your body can comfortably handle, and don't try to support someone else's weight when your own body is in a weak position.

Always follow through with your adjustment; don't quit halfway through and walk off. Always make your efforts a positive experience for your fellow student or partner. Give encouragement and support throughout and after the adjustment. Communicate with your partner so you're in touch with his or her abilities and limitations.

Adjusting the Bow Posture

This Yoga adjustment for the Bow Posture gives you some relaxing benefits that you aren't able to achieve on your own. This adjustment opens your chest and creates flexibility in your shoulders and thighs. This posture is relaxing and refreshing, because you don't have to put much effort into maintaining the pose.

Bow can be problematic for people with lumbar problems. Engaging your abdominal muscles helps stabilize the lower back and prevent overarching.

Before you begin this (or any Yoga adjustment), you and your partner should decide who will do the posture and who will do the adjustments. You can rotate these roles. of course, as you work through multiple repetitions of the exercises. The following steps address the partner doing the posture as the *student* and the Yoga adjuster as, well, the *Yoga adjuster!*

1. **The student begins by lying face down on the floor, with arms extended close to both sides and palms facing upward.**

2. **The student turns his or her head to the side and relaxes for a few breaths, with eyes closed.**

3. **The student bends his or her knees upward at a 90-degree angle and waits for the Yoga adjuster's help.**

4. **The Yoga adjuster sits in a squatting position right behind the student, places his or her feet up under the student's knees, and reaches forward with both hands to take hold of the student's wrists.**

   The student should grasp the Yoga adjuster's wrists as well.

5. **The Yoga adjuster leans back very gently and lifts the student's torso off the floor.**

   The Yoga adjuster doesn't need to lift the student very high for this adjustment to be effective, so both of you should take it easy. This is a mild stretch, and the Yoga adjuster should keep it that way.

6. **As the Yoga adjuster lifts the student upward, the student's knees will gently push the adjuster's feet toward his or her head.**

   Don't let this pushing action go too far; the adjuster's lower legs should remain vertical to the floor (see Figure 21-1).

7. **Hold this pose for five slow, deep breaths (both the adjuster and the student should practice Yoga breathing); then, as the Yoga adjuster takes a final exhalation, he or she lowers the student slowly to the floor.**

8. **Trade places, and repeat Steps 1–7.**

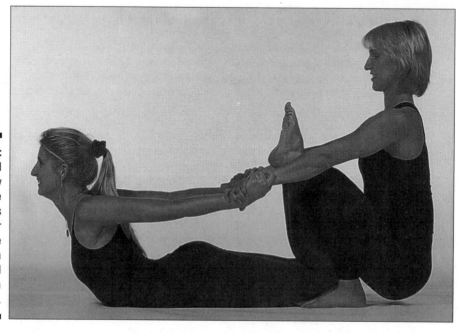

Figure 21-1: This mild Bow Posture stretch is good for both the Yoga student and the Yoga adjuster.

Adjusting the Downward Facing Dog

This Yoga adjustment for the Downward Facing Dog (see the Cheat Sheet) takes the weight off your arms and shoulders because it allows you to really lengthen your entire spine and relax. Although the posture is wonderful in its standard form, it's next to impossible to get the same effect on your own that you achieve with the adjustment I show you in this section.

You need a partner to work through these steps with you. And for this adjustment, you should work with someone who feels comfortable in the Downward Facing Dog. The following steps address the partner doing the posture as the *student* and the Yoga adjuster as the *Yoga adjuster:*

1. **The student goes into the standard Downward Facing Dog Posture.**

2. **The Yoga adjuster stands behind the student, facing the student's back, and places his or her hands on the student's lower back or hips, taking a strong stance — as if ready to push a heavy load.**

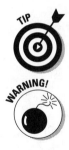

It really helps to have both people on mats.

3. **The Yoga adjuster pushes back and up on the student's hip or lower back.**

   The adjuster's hands should be on the *sacrum,* a bony triangle below the waist, and *never* on the spine itself.

   The Yoga adjuster and student should practice slow, deep breathing, and the student should relax for five complete breaths.

   The Yoga adjuster should ask the student if he or she wants the adjuster to push harder or more lightly at this point. Both partners should communicate throughout the posture to make sure that both are comfortable and secure in the movements.

4. **At the end of the student's fifth complete breath, the Yoga adjuster removes his or her hands from the student and the student relaxes into the Child's Pose (see the Cheat Sheet) for a few complete Yoga breaths.**

5. **Trade places, and follow Steps 1 through 4.**

Practicing Partner Yoga

Partner Yoga is different in some ways from Yoga adjustments, and in other ways, the two are very similar. The reasons that people practice partner Yoga are different than the reasons that draw folks to Yoga adjustments. Practicing partner Yoga is mostly about having fun with your practice and forming beautiful postures with a friend. Partner Yoga is also a great way to stay motivated and directed in your practice. And having someone to help you work through a difficult pose or to help you keep your balance when you're learning a complicated new posture is always helpful.

In the sections that follow, I show you two of my favorite partner Yoga poses. But with a little imagination, you may find that almost any Yoga posture can be a partner posture. The ideal way to practice partner Yoga is to make it a part of a balanced, varied Power Yoga workout program. That way, you're building your skills in individual practice and benefiting from occasional partner practice, all at the same time.

The object of your partner Yoga is to have fun and enjoy a creative, beautiful Power Yoga practice. Don't sacrifice life and limb just to achieve a good partner exercise. Try to work within your own levels of practice — don't think that together, two beginners equal an intermediate or advanced capability! As you do poses with your partner, try to maintain correct alignment of your Yoga posture and remember to breathe and relax. Don't push it: Coordinate and work together with your partner, and have fun.

Howdy, partner!

Partner Yoga is a beautiful and fun way to enjoy Power Yoga with a good friend. Having fun with your practice is a great way to remain excited about Power Yoga, and it's good for your development as a Yoga student. If you and your partner let yourselves be free and creative, you can think of many ways to make your sessions more entertaining and productive. Try playing music that you both enjoy during the session, and see if you can develop routines that create a Power Yoga dance. A really special treat is to travel with your partner to a beautiful outdoor location and enjoy a partners Power Yoga session in Nature's studio. Have a good time with partner Yoga — it's just another way that Yoga brings a soothing touch of love and good feeling into your life.

Partnering with the Standing Downward Dog

In this partner exercise, you do a variation of the Downward Facing Dog Posture (discussed in Chapter 12) in a standing position. This partner posture is a great way to release stress and tension from your shoulders, expand your chest, and create a beautiful bond of energy with your partner.

Both partners follow these steps to achieve the Downward Facing Dog:

1. **Face your partner.**

2. **Extend your arms out straight, and touch each other's palms, with your fingers pointing upward.**

3. **Lift your arms upward as you lower your torso toward the floor and push your hips backward.**

   Think of the traditional Downward Facing Dog posture, and this pose will come easily to you.

4. **Open your chest and shoulders as you arch your back and gaze toward your partner's face.**

   See Figure 21-2.

5. **Hold this position for five slow, deep breaths, and then come back to a standing position and relax.**

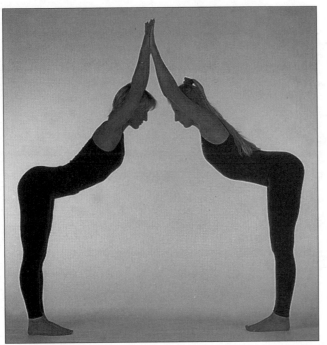

Figure 21-2:
The partners version of Downward Facing Dog releases tension in both partners' neck and shoulders.

Going Boating with your buddy

This is a fun way to practice the Boat Posture, which I explain in Chapter 11, with a partner. This partner posture helps you develop a strong, straight back as it stretches your tight hamstrings.

Both partners follow these steps to achieve the Boat Posture:

1. **Sit on the floor facing each other with your knees bent and toes touching.**

2. **Take hold of your partner's hands or wrists, and flex your feet upward, with the bottoms of your feet touching the bottoms of your partner's feet.**

   Straighten your legs at the same time and try to find a balance between you.

3. **Mold your feet to your partner's feet, and relax for five slow, deep breaths.**

   See Figure 21-3.

4. **Lower your feet to the floor, and release your grip.**

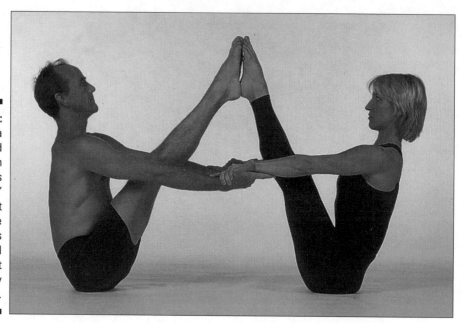

Figure 21-3:
To get a good balance in this partners' Boat Posture, the partners must mold their feet tightly together.

Chapter 22

Fueling Your Yoga Body

*P*ower Yoga is all about burning up calories as you build energy, but your body needs high-powered fuel to keep your big wheels turning throughout your Power Yoga workout. The old saying, "you are what you eat," is never more true than when it's applied to a Power Yoga student. You need nourishment to burn, baby, burn!

In this chapter, I outline a basic healthy, highly nutritious diet. This diet is founded on traditional Yoga principles of food classifications, and it embraces philosophies that date back thousands of years. But that doesn't mean the recipes I give you in this chapter are stale! Here, I share some of my favorite "how to's" for whipping up tasty dishes for breakfast, lunch, and dinner. I even throw in some of my favorite recipes for high-powered, all-natural energy drinks and smoothies. So tie on your napkin and step right up to the Power Yoga health bar and buffet — and don't forget your appetite!

Improving Your Diet for All the Right Reasons

Hippocrates said, "Let your food be your remedies and your remedies be your foods. Build your temple with a strong foundation, and shelter the sacred mind."

Don't be surprised if, after you develop a regular Power Yoga practice, you begin to feel the need to improve your diet. As your body becomes stronger through Power Yoga practice, you may find that you no longer want as much junk food because your body and your mind are drawn to healthier, more nutritious foods. You may choose an apple instead of a chocolate bar and a salad instead of French fries. These changes aren't hard to make; they simply happen over time. Like any machine, your body needs clean, nourishing fuel. Improving your diet is a great way to go beyond merely practicing Yoga and into living Power Yoga. After all, you have a fresh start. Make the most of it!

As you cleanse your body with Yoga postures, you begin to appreciate cleaner foods — those free of chemicals and pesticides. When you choose these foods, you do your part to cut down on pollution and make the world a cleaner, more fertile place. You link your diet to nature, too — taking care of the environment is closely linked with taking care of *you* through a better, more natural diet.

Think of your diet as an evolutionary process. After all, you probably don't eat exactly the same foods that you enjoyed as a kid. As you age, your tastes tend to mature and become more refined. As your body becomes stronger and more flexible, it craves the foods best suited to nourish that kind of natural development.

As your diet continues to evolve, you find yourself eating more whole foods and fewer processed foods. Whole foods, such as an apple, come the way they grew. Processed foods are often unrecognizable imitations of some natural food — such as Cinnamon Apple Sugar-Coated Breakfast Crunchy Chunks (with marshmallows!). When you lead a Power Yoga lifestyle, you also eat lots of raw vegetables and fruits because you draw the most nutrition from foods in their most natural state.

A Quick Guide to Nutrition Basics

Nutrition is the process of supplying proper nourishment (or fuel) to your body. To get the highest quality performance from your body, you need to fuel it with the best possible nutrition. As a Power Yoga practitioner, you're engaged in an athletic lifestyle, so proper nutrition takes on even more importance as you make more demands of your body.

Many people have made the mistake of thinking that their body performs well on junk food. Didn't get enough sleep? Have an extra cup of coffee! Gotta stay up late studying? Eat a bag of chocolate-covered peanuts! Although you can keep ticking right along for a while on a diet of artificially stimulating junk food, you ultimately pay the price for the so-called short-term benefits it brings.

Life is full of choices: You can pick your own path and make your own decisions. When it comes to fueling your body, though, you shouldn't cut corners. Power Yoga is one of the highest quality forms of exercise, so if you want to put out perfect energy, you need to fuel your body with the highest quality fuel available. If you plant a garden in bad, thin soil, the crops won't be healthy and strong. If you feed your body junk food, you're limiting your performance potential and asking for health problems — and sooner or later, you'll get them.

Putting together nutrition's building blocks

People haven't yet entered the space age eating patterns predicted by the science fiction shows of the 1950s and 1960s. In the kitchens of yesterday's tomorrows, folks just popped a breakfast pill or slowly savored a lunch chip, and miraculously, all their nutritional needs had been met, without cutting, cleaning, peeling — or enjoying — a thing. The pop-a-pill meal didn't happen, thank goodness, and most people are stuck with enjoying good food to fill their stomachs and their nutritional needs.

When you consider the complexity of the human body, your nutritional needs are relatively simple. Your body requires these nutritional elements:

- ✔ **Carbohydrates:** For energy and to maintain proper blood sugar
- ✔ **Fats:** To supply your body with energy, fuel, and warmth
- ✔ **Minerals:** To build tissue and serve as body regulators
- ✔ **Protein:** To build and repair your body cell tissues
- ✔ **Vitamins:** To maintain your body's normal metabolic functions

Each of these elements is available in a number of forms, and choosing the sources of these elements is another important part of maintaining a healthy, well-balanced diet — see the following section.

Yoga food categories

In traditional Yoga philosophy, all foods fall into one of three main categories:

✔ **Satwic food:** Healthy, wholesome, nourishing food that supplies your body with all necessary ingredients for a healthy, active life.

✔ **Rajasic food:** Food, such as sugar and coffee, that unnaturally stimulates your body, causing you to go beyond your normal capabilities. Overtaxing your system with this kind of poorly powered body can cause much strain and depletion to both your mental and physical condition.

✔ **Tamasic food:** Eating just plain unhealthy food, such as fried food, junk food, and red meat, detracts from your health and creates an environment for sickness and disease.

Finding the right food sources

To keep your body active and healthy, a balanced diet needs to provide the right quantities of all the elements listed in the preceding section. But how much is enough, and in what form should you consume these nutritional building blocks? This list is a quick guide to some of the most common nutritional sources:

✔ **Carbohydrates:** Carbohydrates occur in two forms — simple and complex.

- *Simple carbohydrates* are sugars, found in cane sugar, lactose (from milk), and maltose (from malt). Try to limit your intake of simple carbohydrates, because they are processed very quickly into your body's bloodstream as sugar and, as a result, tend to undermine your body's natural metabolism.

- *Complex carbohydrates,* found in grains, fruits, and vegetables, transform into sugar more slowly within your system, so they don't give your metabolism the "sugar jolt" of simple carbs.

✔ **Fats:** As much as you hear about low-fat and nonfat foods today, fat is an essential part of the human diet. It's only when you take in excessive *saturated fats* — from meat, dairy, and heated oils — that you harm your body and upset your nutritional balance. Animal fats come from meat and dairy products and tend to be high in saturated fat (the bad kind of fat) and cholesterol. Carefully monitor your intake of animal fats — if you choose to consume them at all. Most cold pressed, unheated vegetable fats are *unsaturated,* and they come from such sources as nuts, seeds, avocadoes, olives, and selected other fruits and vegetables.

✔ **Proteins:** You can divide proteins into two broad categories — animal protein and plant protein.

- *Animal protein* is found in meat, dairy products, and eggs.

- *Plant protein* is found in beans, legumes, seeds, nuts, seaweed, bee pollen, and spirulina (you find out more about bee pollen, spirulina, and other natural food supplements in the section "Scoping out super food supplements," later in this chapter).

Your body can assimilate both kinds of protein, so you can choose to eat one form of protein, or both.

✔ **Vitamins and minerals:** These are available to you in fruits, vegetables, nuts, seeds, beans, legumes, grains, seaweed, bee pollen, and spirulina (see the section "Scoping out super food supplements," later in this chapter). Some people believe that your body requires vitamins and minerals from animal products as well, but scientific evidence doesn't support that notion. I personally haven't used meat, dairy products, or eggs for over 30 years, and I'm an active and extremely healthy person.

Balancing cholesterol, fat, and fiber

Fats come in both saturated and unsaturated forms. Saturated fats are the most harmful to your health, and they have been linked to hardening of the arteries, heart disease, and obesity. Most animal fats are saturated and contain high levels of cholesterols that develop into artery-clogging plaque. Most vegetable fats are unsaturated and contain good cholesterol that actually helps keep arteries clear and healthy. (Fried and roasted fats — even vegetable fats — are bad news, though, so steer clear.) Although avocados and raw nuts contain fats, you're unlikely to ever build up unhealthy levels of cholesterol eating these foods.

Fiber is an important cleansing tool for your body. Fiber helps absorb and eliminate fats from your system, and it helps to sweep out your intestinal tract and keep it in proper working order. If your diet lacks natural fiber, your intestinal tract can't function properly, and as a result, your health will suffer. The highest fiber foods are fruits, vegetables, whole grains, legumes, nuts, and flaxseed.

Scoping out super food supplements

You can't build a nutrition plan around food supplements. You have to eat good, healthy foods and maintain a balanced blend of nutrition from a number of sources. But if you feel that even your healthy diet choices still don't supply adequate amounts of certain food elements, try adding some nutritional supplements to your diet.

You can find plenty of high-quality multivitamin supplements at your local health food store. The natural food supplements listed in this section can make a big difference in building a balanced, healthy diet.

People can have different reactions to different foods, and you may find that you have an allergic reaction to a new food substance or supplement. Go easy when trying any new food supplement until you determine that you're not exhibiting any allergic symptoms or other negative reactions.

- **Bee pollen:** A wonderful high-energy food supplement. These tiny granules are packed full of vitamins and amino acids. Even a teaspoon or less of bee pollen, taken just before and after workouts, can give you a strong, healthy energy boost. You can mix bee pollen granules in a fruit drink or take it in capsule form.

- **Spirulina and blue-green algae:** A freshwater algae proven to be one of the most nutritious dried plant foods available. If you could take any kind of food to a deserted island, this would be it. Spirulina and blue-green algae are very high in proteins that your body can easily assimilate. This food also contains chlorophyll (the green pigment in plants) and a long list of amino acids and vitamins.

- **Seaweeds:** Natural food sources from the ocean that are high in minerals and are a source of natural iodine. Many authorities have found seaweeds to help remove radioactive particles and heavy metals from your body. Seaweeds come in a variety of forms, and you can use them as seasoning, in soups and salads, or as a supplement.

- **Wheat grass:** A highly nutritious fresh food that offers one of the highest sources of chlorophyll found in any food. Wheat grass is usually available as a juice; it's made from ten-day-old sprouted wheat, from which the juices have been extracted. You can drink an ounce or two of wheat grass juice straight or mixed with other juices. Get your wheat grass juice fresh-squeezed from your local health store or juice bar.

I'm aware that you can find plenty of unhealthy dietary supplements on the store shelves — drinks, powders, candies, and pills that guarantee to build your energy while helping you to lose weight. As in most areas of life, though, good nutrition doesn't come from a simple and easy-to-use magic bullet. Food supplements and energy boosters should come from nature and serve as merely a small part of a healthy, balanced diet.

Building a better diet

If you feel that your diet isn't quite what it should be, don't despair! You can build a better diet without going to extremes. In fact, extreme and dramatic dietary changes tend to backfire because your body has to ease into any kind of change. So rather than throwing out all the food in your pantry and starting from scratch, take the following common-sense steps to make incremental improvements in your current eating habits:

- ✔ Add more fiber to your diet.
- ✔ Cut down on saturated fat.
- ✔ Avoid junk food.
- ✔ Cut back on meat and dairy products.
- ✔ Add more fresh fruits and vegetables to your diet.
- ✔ Add more raw uncooked fruits and vegetables.
- ✔ Drink plenty of water, fruit, and vegetable juices daily.

Keep improving your diet over time, and eventually, you'll end up eating a well-balanced, healthy, nutritional mix of foods. But remember that you don't develop your eating habits overnight, and you can't change them that quickly, either. Be attentive to what you're eating and think about the impact it has on your body. By eating with purpose — just as you move through your Power Yoga routines with intent and purpose — you are naturally drawn to nutritious, healthy foods.

Fueling Up throughout the Day

In this section, I share my favorite recipes for some of the best natural energy drinks that you can make using fresh-squeezed fruit and vegetable juices, homemade nut milks, and powerful bee pollen boosters. I also offer some tried-and-true recipes for breakfast, lunch, and dinner. And I don't forget dessert!

If possible, buy fresh, organically grown ingredients for these recipes; you'll get more of a "health bang" for your investment of time and energy in preparing these healthy dishes.

Manoa's Green Heaven

When I first got interested in health, I met a really interesting woman at a local health food store. Her name was Manoa, and she was always energetic and in the best of spirits; I never saw her in a bad mood. Manoa told me that her secret to a healthy, active, long life was this wonderful, natural energy drink.

Tools: *Juicer*

Preparation time: *5 minutes*

Yield: *One serving*

4 leaves romaine lettuce	*3 stalks celery, quartered*
1 small bunch spinach	*2 large apples, cored*
1 small bunch parsley	*Fresh mint leaf to taste*
Dandelion greens to taste	

1 One at a time, roll the romaine lettuce, spinach, parsley, and dandelion greens into a tight ball and push them through the juicer.

2 Push the celery and apple through the juicer; garnish with mint (optional but good!).

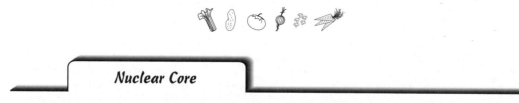

Nuclear Core

The name of this recipe makes you want to get up and run for cover, but you'll be dancing for joy when you try this exotic, nutritious, warming brew.

Tools: *Juicer*

Preparation time: *5 minutes*

Yield: *One serving*

1-inch square fresh ginger	*Dash cayenne pepper*
5 leaves romaine lettuce	*3 stalks celery, quartered*
4 carrots, quartered	

1 Push the ginger, romaine lettuce, and celery through the juicer.

Using the celery to push the greens through the juicer not only makes your juicing job easier, but the celery helps you get more juice out of the lettuce.

2 Juice the carrots, and add the cayenne pepper.

Purple People Power

This drink has a rich, dark purple color due to the fresh beet juice. The vitamin-rich greens and the protein from the pumpkin seeds help this colorful drink deliver a high-energy boost.

Tools: *Blender, juicer*

Preparation time: *5 minutes*

Yield: *One serving*

⅓ cup raw pumpkin seeds

¼ avocado

1 small bunch spring greens

1 small bunch parsley

1 raw beet

2 carrots, quartered

3 stalks celery, quartered

1 Place the pumpkin seeds and avocado in a blender.

2 Roll the spring greens and parsley into a ball, and push through a juicer, using the celery and carrots to push the greens. Slice the beet, and push through the juicer.

3 Pour half the juice into your blender with the pumpkin seeds and avocado, and blend until creamy smooth. Pour the remaining juice into the blender, and blend briefly.

Sunshine Power House

This drink is sure to brighten your day with vitamin C, protein, and lots of nutrition from bee pollen.

Tools: *Blender*

Preparation time: *5 minutes*

Yield: *One serving*

⅓ cup raw hulled sunflower seeds

½ tablespoon bee pollen

10 ounces fresh-squeezed orange juice, divided

½ ripe frozen banana

4 strawberries

1 Place sunflower seeds, bee pollen, 5 ounces of orange juice, and the half banana in a blender; blend until creamy smooth.

2 Add remaining orange juice and strawberries; blend until smooth.

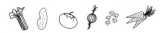

Patanjali's Paradise

For such a natural, healthy drink, this smoothie tastes truly decadent. Enjoy this treat without feeling guilty or worrying that you're damaging your good health. It's as good for you as it is good!

Freezing the banana before using it helps to make this smoothie creamier.

Tools: *Small bowl, blender, juicer*

Preparation time: *5 minutes*

Freezing/Soaking time: *8 hours*

Yield: *One serving*

3 unsulphured, organic dried black figs	*⅓ cup almonds*
6 ounces purified water	*1 apple, cored*
1 ripe banana, peeled and frozen	

1 Place the figs in a small container and completely cover the figs with the water. Soak overnight. Remove figs from the water, and set water aside.

2 Place fig water, banana, and almonds in a blender; blend until creamy.

3 Cut stems off figs, and place in blender. Blend until smooth.

4 Juice the apple. Pour apple juice into the blender with all the remaining ingredients, and blend until smooth.

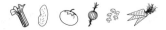

Wholesome, Hot Wheat Cereal

Instead of the usual whatever-pops-out-of-the-toaster breakfast, try this healthy hot cereal dish and see how good you feel. You can find whole wheat berries at any natural foods store and many grocery stores. If you have trouble locating them, substitute any variety of grain available. You may also substitute other nuts or fruits for the almonds and apple called for here.

Tools: *Pot or large saucepan, blender*

Preparation time: *5 minutes*

Yield: *One serving*

1 cup whole wheat berries

2 cups water

⅓ cup raw almonds

½ cored apple

1 banana, divided

Water to taste

Honey to taste

1 Place wheat berries and water in a saucepan. Bring to a boil, turn the heat down to a low setting, cover the pan, and let simmer for 30–45 minutes, or until the grain has absorbed the water.

2 In a blender, grind the almonds, apple, and ½ the banana, adding a small amount of water (just enough for the mixture to blend smoothly).

3 Pour the blended fruit and nut sauce over the cooked wheat, and slice the other banana half on top; sweeten to taste with honey.

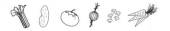

Powerfully Good Lunch

Instead of running out for a fast-food lunch, try making this tasty sandwich to take for your lunch. Bring along celery sticks stuffed with your favorite natural nut butter and honey to enjoy with this sandwich. You'll return to your afternoon's work full of energy.

Tools: *Two bowls, toaster*

Preparation time: *10 minutes*

Yield: *One serving*

3 or 4 strips dulse seaweed

6 ounces baked tofu

1 avocado, divided

3 tablespoons apple cider vinegar

Juice of ½ lemon

2 slices sprouted whole-grain bread

Vegetables of your choice (alfalfa sprouts, lettuce, onion, tomato, and so on)

1 Place seaweed in a bowl, and cover with water to rehydrate. As the seaweed sits, slice the tofu into a few thin slices.

2 In another bowl, mash ½ the avocado with the vinegar and lemon juice to create an avocado mayonnaise. Toast the bread lightly and spread the avocado mayonnaise on both bread slices.

3 Place the sliced baked tofu, seaweed, the other ½ avocado, and raw vegetables, between the bread slices, and enjoy.

Guru's Millet and Veggies in Carrot Sauce

Try out this tasty, low-fat, high-energy dinner. It will leave you feeling satisfied and energized.

Tools: *Two large saucepans, blender*

Preparation time: *20 minutes*

Yield: *One serving*

3 cups water	*⅓ cup hulled sunflower seeds*
1 cup millet	*2 tablespoons flaxseed*
1 teaspoon sea salt	*2 tablespoons tamari*
½ bunch broccoli	*Water to cover*
2 carrots	*8 ounces fresh carrot juice*
1 yellow squash	

1 Place water, millet, and salt into a saucepan. Bring to a boil; reduce heat to medium or low, and cook for about 40 minutes or until the water is gone.

2 Break broccoli into good size chunks, and slice carrots and squash. In a separate pot, lightly steam broccoli and carrots; add the squash and steam for a few minutes more.

3 Place sunflower seeds and flaxseeds in a blender; add the tamari and just enough water to cover them. Juice the carrots and add the juice to the blender and blend until creamy smooth. This is the carrot sauce.

4 Pour the carrot sauce over the cooked millet, and top with the remaining steamed vegetables. Serve with salad and whole-grain garlic bread.

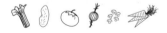

Mango Tango Dessert

Dessert need not be loaded with refined sugar and fat to be enjoyable and easy to make. Try this simple and tasty alternative to gelatin or pudding — your body will be glad you did.

Tools: *Blender*

Preparation time: *5 minutes*

Yield: *One serving*

1 ripe mango	*2 tablespoons flaxseed*
½ ripe banana	*2 tablespoons water*
½ ripe avocado	*Parsley or mint sprigs*
Orange slices	

Place all ingredients except orange slices and parsley or mint in a blender, and blend until creamy smooth. Serve in small desert cups; garnish each with ½ an orange slice and parsley or mint.

Part VI
The Part of Tens

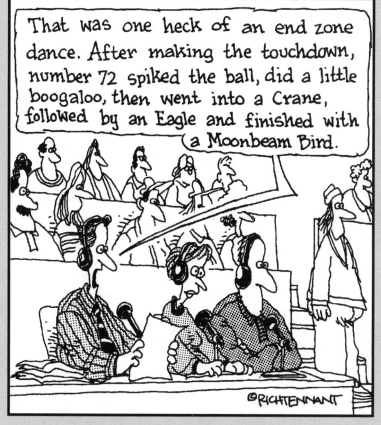

The 5th Wave By Rich Tennant

That was one heck of an end zone dance. After making the touchdown, number 72 spiked the ball, did a little boogaloo, then went into a Crane, followed by an Eagle and finished with a Moonbeam Bird.

©RICHTENNANT

In this part . . .

These short, and I like to think sweet, chapters give you my secrets for making the most of your Power Yoga practice, some motivation tips, and my favorite places to practice in Mother Nature's studio.

Chapter 23

Ten Reasons to Turn On Your Power

In This Chapter

▶ Losing weight while building strength and flexibility

▶ Building a stronger, more organized mind

▶ Enjoying the whole-body benefits of regular Power Yoga practice

Sometimes, you just need a little nudge to get you to practice your Power Yoga. I used to have some problems with procrastination. If I had a particularly tiring day at my job, I'd come home and think, "I'm just too tired to work out tonight — I've had enough exercise for one day, anyway." Well, I soon discovered that my Yoga routine was just what I needed to refresh myself after a hard day's work. I just had to get over that momentary mental resistance — something I compare to a tired, sleepy kid refusing to go to bed. Sometimes, your head doesn't want to give your body what it needs.

When your head starts screaming, "But I don't *want* to," remind yourself of all the reasons you *do* want your Power Yoga workout. The benefits of Power Yoga are endless, but in this chapter, I list my top ten favorite reasons to love Power Yoga. Use this list as your inspiration, or create your own!

Losing Weight is Easier

When you practice Power Yoga, you work your muscles, you sweat, and you breathe hard. In other words, practicing Power Yoga burns calories and helps you lose weight. The more you practice, the more pounds and inches you lose. I know a lot of people who have been amazed at how much weight they lost and how quickly they lost it after beginning a Power Yoga practice.

Power Yoga workouts leave you feeling energetic, so you may not realize just how strenuous your workout is. Deep, slow Yoga breathing combined with the fluid movement of your Power Yoga exercises helps you power through even high-level routines. You lose weight and feel great — a prime reason to get off the couch and onto your Yoga mat.

You Get Stronger

Most people don't associate Yoga with beefing up muscle mass. But Power Yoga is one of the best methods known for strengthening muscles. You can understand why weight lifting is a good muscle-building activity. Well, Power Yoga is actually a form of weightlifting; throughout your workout, you're lifting and moving the weight of your body. Through powerful exercises and fluid, connecting movements (or *vinyasas*), you build muscle strength, balance, and coordination.

You Become More Flexible

Power Yoga increases flexibility in your joints, muscles, and connective tissue. The stretching and counter-stretching movements of any good Power Yoga routine help you maintain balanced progress in your quest for increased strength and flexibility. Power Yoga offers a safe and effective way to increase your flexibility because it works all your major joints and muscle groups. Though your practice builds your strength, you don't need to worry about becoming muscle bound from regular Power Yoga practice. Your body makes equal gains in flexibility *and* strength from your workouts.

Relaxation is Built In

For 5,000 years, people have been using Yoga as a technique for releasing stress and tension. Power Yoga, though newer than the more traditional Yoga forms, may be one of the best forms for attaining deep relaxation.

Yoga is a powerful relaxation technique for a couple of reasons:

- ✔ Slow, deep, synchronized breathing helps send oxygen through your system and relaxes tense muscles.
- ✔ Yoga postures stretch and counter-stretch your muscles, working to loosen muscles *and* strengthen them at the same time. Power Yoga brings opposing pairs of muscles into balance and harmony.

Add to those traditional Yoga features the fluid, graceful movements of the connecting movements of Power Yoga, and you've put together a powerful prescription for a soothing, relaxing workout. The deep relaxation that caps every Power Yoga routine reinforces the calming benefits of the practice and gives you a soothing touch of relaxation that stays with you for hours.

You Free Your Mind

All the powerful relaxation that Power Yoga brings doesn't mean that you spend your days sitting around contemplating your navel and thinking, "Wow, man, this is cool." One of Power Yoga's main benefits is its ability to help you think more clearly. Because your body is growing healthier and stronger, you have more energy. Your deep, powerful Yoga breathing sends big, healthy supplies of oxygenated blood through your body, improving your circulatory system and clearing your head. And regular Power Yoga practice teaches you self-discipline (though the lessons tend to be painless). You become calmer, and as a result, more organized. Your mind becomes more disciplined and your thought processes more orderly.

You Gain Self-Confidence

As you advance through your practice and become a regular Power Yoga practitioner, your self-confidence soars. You look better, feel better, and have more energy — you even seem to have more time in your day. As a result, you feel strong, comfortable, and confident. The self-confidence you gain from regular Power Yoga practice can serve you in everything you do — from getting that new job to resolving family issues you may have been avoiding. The more comfortable you are in your body, the more comfortable you are in your mind. Confidence feeds itself, so you just continue to feel better as your practice matures — another great reason to say "Yes" to Power Yoga!

You Create a Mind–Body Connection

Many exercises pump up your body, but few fitness programs feed your body *and* your mind like Power Yoga does. When you start practicing Power Yoga postures, you don't just discover where to put your hands or how to position your feet. Power Yoga is all about balance, and the wonderful balance of a strong mind–body connection runs through every breath, posture, and *vinyasa* of a Power Yoga routine. In Power Yoga, you're encouraged to be aware of everything you do and think about every movement you make. Your body and mind begin to work more closely together, and the resulting strong body–mind connection makes you function with more clarity, stability, and assurance in everything you do.

You Build Total Body Fitness

Most exercises target specific skills or build selected muscle groups. Bicycling, for example, strengthens your legs and develops endurance. Dancing builds coordination and offers aerobic training, and weightlifting targets building muscle mass. Power Yoga, on the other hand, offers all of these benefits and a whole lot more. Regular Power Yoga practice gives your entire body a balanced, strength-training workout; it builds endurance; it develops flexibility, balance, and coordination; it relaxes your muscles and your mind; and it burns calories through strong aerobic training. All in all, you can't find a better whole-body workout than the one you get from a good Power Yoga practice.

You Become Successful

Regular Power Yoga practice leaves you feeling strong, confident, and full of energy. You become more focused, have greater mental clarity, and an increased physical confidence. Power Yoga helps you channel that energy into making a better life. You become more in touch with the world around you, you see things with greater clarity, and you focus your attention and energies on things that matter. You begin to put things in their proper perspective and recognize real priorities instead of accepting the conventional wisdom. Whether you're a candlestick maker, garbage collector, stockbroker, or the President of the United States (or even the author of a ...For Dummies book), Power Yoga can help you be happier and more successful at whatever you do.

Being a Yogi or Yogini is Just Plain Cool

Imagine yourself at a cocktail party — everyone's standing around nibbling food off of toothpicks and downing martinis. Someone comes up to you and says, "I run, ride bikes, swim, and play golf. What do you do?" You take another sip of your sparkling water, swallow that last mouthful of almonds, and say, "I do Power Yoga, friend." A silence descends on the room, replaced by the awed murmurs of the impressed crowd. You hear, "Wow, now there is a way totally cool person!" and you realize that they're talking about *you!* Power Yoga is becoming more popular all the time, and being a yogi or yogini sure has more cachet than slogging away at the fitness center or running marathons in the rain. So come over to the cool side, and join the Power set.

Chapter 24

Ten Secrets for Mastering Power Yoga

*T*o really excel in your Power Yoga practice, you must be humble, have a positive attitude, and discover your connection with the energy you call *life*. Anyone can practice Power Yoga, have a great time in the process, and enjoy the many benefits of a regular practice. But if you want to gain the most from Power Yoga and savor the true essence of this ancient and magical system, you need to keep a few key words of wisdom in mind. If I had known then what I know now, my early years in Yoga practice would have gone much more smoothly. In this chapter, I offer some sage advice and hard-earned wisdom to help ease your path toward yogic enlightenment. Read and become wiser, grasshopper.

Be Humble

Don't fight your Yoga practice: Don't try to control it, overcome it, or conquer it. You have to relax to find the connecting energy that runs through life. Humble yourself in the face of this powerful system and work with your Power Yoga, not against it. Take it slow and easy. Don't be competitive (with yourself or anyone else), and approach your practice with an open mind. Let your mind flow through your practice, and your body will follow. Respect the energy your body generates during practice and think of it as part of the energy of all life. Remembering this connection can make your practice more powerful — and more fulfilling.

Have Patience

If you rush through your Power Yoga practice, don't expect to gain anything but a load of stress. Enough of your life is hectic and fast-paced; you don't need to add a stress-filled rush-rush Power Yoga practice to your schedule. Finishing first may be important in other aspects of your life, but your Power Yoga practice needs to be an exception to the norm.

Practice patience as you practice Yoga. Don't expect to accomplish everything the first day. If you practice regularly and moderately, your body responds more quickly than it does if you push it. If you practice patience and moderation, you succeed every time you sit down on your mat to enjoy a quality practice.

Practice with Love and Compassion

Focus your mind on peaceful, loving thoughts and embrace a compassionate outlook as you do your Yoga practice. I'm talking about having love and compassion for the entire practice of Yoga. To gain the most from your practice, you really have to love to do it and be compassionate toward yourself. Don't force yourself to do your practice; wait until you want to do it, and then let it become your passion.

Power Yoga can be something very special — something that you look forward to and love. Think of every practice as a vacation. Use your practice as a means of developing love and compassion for everyone and everything that shares your planet.

Cross-Train

Although Power Yoga is a complete fitness system, you can benefit by cross-training with other physical activities as well. I firmly believe that if you want to succeed in Power Yoga, you need to practice non-Power Yoga activities, too. You can take long walks, dance, practice other forms of Yoga, participate in group sports, work in your garden, or incorporate any of your favorite physical activities into your regular fitness schedule. You don't have to practice Power Yoga every day without any breaks. Be balanced in your approach to fitness — enjoy your life and be as active as you can — and your Power Yoga will benefit. You'll look forward to your practice, have fewer injuries in your more active pursuits, and find ways to use your Yoga techniques in the other physical activities you enjoy.

Respect Your Limits

You have a unique body. Because everyone is put together a little differently, some folks have a harder time with certain activities than others. This truth carries over to practicing Power Yoga postures. No one is perfect at every Yoga posture, and you won't be, either. But don't let that get you down. Natural limitations are the reasons we use Yoga props and practice Yoga adjustments. Don't ever try to push yourself into doing a posture just because you think that you *should* be able to do it, or because that older woman beside you can do it. The true yogi or yogini knows his or her limits and works with those limits — not against them.

Listen to your body, and stop when it tells you to stop. Rest when it says it needs rest. Try to grow in your practice, but don't ever try to force your body into doing something that it doesn't want to do. An injury only adds to your physical limitations.

Be Clear on Your Goals

Now, if your goal in practicing Power Yoga is just to relax and release a little stress and tension, that's fine. If your goal is to develop a lot of strength and flexibility, that's fine, too. But you need to be clear on what your goals are if you want to achieve them. If you want to practice at the highest level, you have to be clear about that goal, and you need to visualize yourself achieving it. As you practice, just keep telling yourself, "I know I can do this. I can accomplish this level of practice."

If you're practicing just to relax, keep that goal in mind, and remember not to allow yourself to become impatient with the pace or angry with yourself for not mastering a posture. When you practice with a specific goal in mind, your practice is more productive, directed, and beneficial in every way.

Visualize Your Success

Before you actually move into a Yoga posture, visualize yourself moving into the posture. When your mind flows into the posture this way, your body will follow. Positive visualization is a technique used by many great athletes, and it's a strong tool for Power Yoga students, as well. *Remember:* Think positive thoughts and visualize yourself accomplishing what you're going to do before you actually do it. This process can benefit your Power Yoga practice as well as any other task you undertake in your daily life.

Relax and Rest

If you want to succeed at building an effective Power Yoga practice, you have to have adequate rest. That means getting enough sleep and taking occasional breaks from your hectic schedule to slow down, enjoy a walk in the park, chat with a neighbor, read a book, or just stare at the world around you. Power Yoga can be a very powerful system, but you limit your body's ability to draw from that power if you limit its rest. Don't ever skip the relaxation exercise at the end of each workout; allow yourself at least 5 and as many as 30 minutes of rest in each deep relaxation session. Relax after each practice, enjoy a little recreation, and get plenty of sleep; that's an important prescription for building a successful Power Yoga practice.

Stoke Your Furnace with Good Nutrition

Okay, eating that sack of donuts won't kill you — today, at least. But you can get away with eating junk food for only so long. Yoga has its roots in nature, and part of succeeding in Power Yoga is becoming one with nature. A big part of being connected to nature is respecting your body. Regular Power Yoga practice demands a lot of your body, and if you want to develop — rather than deplete — your body's resources, you have to give it good fuel. By following a diet of healthy, natural food and large quantities of fresh, pure water, you help your body grow strong and healthy. The fact that you're practicing Power Yoga means that you want to have a healthy body. So don't fight your progress by crippling your body with bad food. (Turn to Chapter 22 for more information — and some recipes — to help fuel your body.)

Never Stop Studying

Notice that I never say, "Eventually, you will master Power Yoga," nor do I refer to anyone as having *perfected* Power Yoga. Instead, I always talk about Power Yoga as a practice because, in reality, it isn't something that you ever finish finding out about — you never absorb everything there is to know about any aspect of Yoga. All yogis and yoginis remain students throughout their lives. And you can benefit from everything and everyone you encounter. Just as the ancient masters based the first Yoga practices on their observations of nature, so can you. You can discover gems by observing your friends, your dog, the stars, and the wind — everything that moves, breathes, or exists on this planet has some connection to the energy of Yoga. It's to your benefit to find these connections wherever you can.

Chapter 25

Ten Great Outdoor Practice Locations

*P*racticing Yoga outdoors is a wonderful experience. But you have to give your outdoor locations some forethought. For example, you probably wouldn't enjoy an outdoor practice in Juneau in January, or in Times Square at just about any time of year. Your outdoor location needs to be relatively clean, quiet, and comfortable if you want to really enjoy a good Power Yoga workout. It also makes sense to check for environmental hazards — stones and other debris under your mat do nothing to enhance your experience. Remember not to look directly at the sun (it's bad for your retinas), and if you're allergic to bees or other stinging insects, make sure that you're prepared in case you get stung.

Practicing outdoors not only gives you the opportunity to get close to nature but also to take advantage of Mother Nature's Yoga-enhancing gifts: sunshine to help you warm up, breezes to keep you moving, and sounds to help you focus — the sound of cicadas can be the om hum of the universe. Under the right conditions, an outdoor workout can bring you hundreds of times the benefit of any indoor practice.

In this chapter, I suggest some of my favorite types of outdoor locations for a good Power Yoga session. These locations can really enhance your practice, and I think that you'll like the ones you try. But you're a creative person — after reading through this list, you can probably come up with plenty of great workout spots that I haven't even thought of. A good outdoor spot doesn't have to be exotic — you may find Power Yoga nirvana in your own back yard!

Powering-Up Your Yoga in the Mountains

Mountains have a wonderful amount of great, clean, quality fresh air (unless you're in one of the mountain top smog capitols of the world, like Mexico City). Practicing your Yoga at a higher altitude is a wonderful treat. The air is a little thinner, so you have to take it easy at first. But mountain air is easy to breathe — it's cooler and feels fresher than the air you're used to. Plus, you get some beautiful views in the mountains.

You can practice at elevations anywhere from 100 feet to 12,000 feet. Just take it easy and make sure that you're acclimated to the air before you begin your practice. Take your Yoga mat so you have a soft, consistent surface and then tap into the power and wisdom of the venerable mountains.

Being a Shade-Tree Yogi

I was raised in the mild climate of southern Texas, so I practiced Yoga outdoors right from the beginning. The summers in Texas get very hot, so I was naturally drawn to the shade of the large oak trees near my home. Practicing in the shade of trees is a powerful and energizing experience. You feel the energy of the mighty tree, you sway with the breeze that blows through its branches, and your Yoga develops a power and rhythm that you never find in a studio.

Rolling in Clover

When you hear songs and poetry written about walking barefoot through clover, you can believe that the singer is talking about a special feeling. Walking through a field and then laying down your blanket and Yoga mat and practicing in the grass is a wonderful, rejuvenating experience. You smell the grass and wildflowers around you, feel the sunshine, hear the birds, and all your senses become alert and in tune with the world around you.

Early evening is the best time to enjoy this type of practice; the sun is low and gentle, and your body can tap into the shifting of light to darkness. After your relaxation exercise, look around you — you may be right next to a four-leaf clover, and you don't want to overlook *that* piece of luck!

Being Mesmerized by the Ocean

The ocean is a very powerful and magnetic place. People have always been drawn to the sea, and that's a good thing, because it covers most of our planet! You can have a powerful and magical Power Yoga experience when you workout near the ocean. Now, you need to be a bit selective here, because the ocean can be less than calming on stormy, windy days. But on quiet mornings, the life of the seaside can add energy and drive to your work-out. The rhythm of the waves, the crying of the gulls, and the wind blowing over the beach all contribute to the movement and *dance* of your Power Yoga routine. If you're lucky enough to be near palm trees, you can get a double boost from working out under their shade. You gain a closer understanding of paradise when you try this workout location.

Drawing Your Power from the Desert

Practicing Yoga in the Mohave may not sound like much fun to you, but in the early morning and evening hours, the desert can be quite cool and accommo-dating. Perch your mat on a high plateau and see some of Nature's most spec-tacular scenery. You're likely to be undisturbed, so you can enjoy a quiet practice that puts you directly in touch with the spirit of the desert.

Embracing Nature in the City

If you can't get away from the city, look for outdoor practice areas near your home. For example, neighborhood, county, or state parks offer wonderful tranquil grounds. I was raised in Houston, Texas, and you can often find me in the local arboretum practicing my Yoga with all the wonderful trees. Another great location is on the grounds of a local college campus. You can even try the porch of your own home. Use your imagination — when this old world starts getting you down, just climb up on your roof and do some Yoga.

Drifting Under the Autumn Trees

Pick a nice location with a good level spot. Place your mat under the trees so you can experience the leaves as they fall. Start practicing your Yoga exer-cise, and as the wind blows, you'll be showered by a rainbow of red, yellow, and orange as the fall leaves dance in the wind and slowly float back down to the earth — raining colors all over you. This memorable experience is one you won't want to forget.

Finding Tranquility in the Forest

If you live near a forest or national park, you have a wonderful setting ready-made for outdoor Power Yoga practice. Find yourself a clear spot in the thick, cool shade of the trees. During your breathing and relaxation exercises, listen to the sound of the birds and the wind moving through the treetops. Breathe in the perfume of the pine needles and the rich black earth on the forest floor. You'll emerge from the forest feeling fresher, more alive, and more at peace than you've ever felt before.

Burying Your Feet in the Mississippi Mud

The banks of a river or stream or the edges of a lake or pond are wonderful places to have a great Power Yoga workout. The air is usually fresh and clear near the water, and any outdoor water source is a prime center of activity for birds and wildlife. Instead of jumping and running when you see insects, mice, and small animals, just keep on working through your routine and try to feel connected to the life teeming around you. (Of course, if a snake crawls on your Yoga mat, you may want to stop moving and hold your breath 'til she goes on her way.) Position yourself where you can hear the soothing sound of water over the rocks. By listening to the water, you can combine softness and strength in your practice.

Clicking Your Heels Together to Find Paradise in Your Own Backyard

And don't forget that the best place to practice Power Yoga may be right in your own backyard. You may have already created one of the best backdrops that you can have for a powerful, peaceful Power Yoga workout. Under your favorite shade tree, on the deck, beside the kids' wading pool — wherever you feel most energized and happy is a good place to be. Try to arrange your workout time when you can be alone and (if possible) unobserved by curious neighbors. But if it's not possible to be totally isolated from the people around you, that's okay, too. Concentrate and focus your energy and attention on the natural sounds and smells around you, and try to ignore the sounds of cars, music from the neighbor's stereo, and your spouse yelling at the kids to stop fighting. Try practicing right at sunset or sunrise, or any time, you can just walk out on the lawn and find a peaceful spot to practice. Set your blanket down and start practicing, and let the rest of the world fade away.

Part VII

Appendixes

The 5th Wave   By Rich Tennant

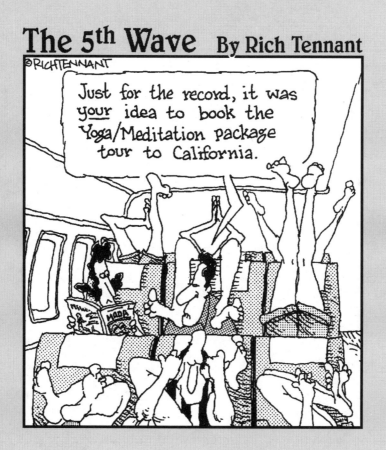

Just for the record, it was your idea to book the Yoga/Meditation package tour to California.

In this part . . .

The language of Yoga is ancient Sanskrit. In Appendix A I give you a basic glossary of the Sanskrit terms and pronunciation for Yoga poses. The second appendix is a guide to Power Yoga–related resources: clothes and other accessories to enhance your practice, books to read, magazines and Web sites to browse, and more.

Appendix A
Yoga Vocabulary

Adho Mukha Svanasana *(ahd-ho mook-hah shvah-nah -sah-nah):* Downward Facing Dog Posture

Akarna *(ar-kah-na):* near or toward the ear

Akarna Dhanurasana *(ar-kah-na dah-nu-rah-sah-nah):* Shooting the Bow Posture

Anga: limbs; the body; a limb or part of the body

Angustha: big toe

Apana *(ah-pah-nah):* downward going life-force

Ardha *(ahrd-ha):* half

Ardha Chandrasana *(ahrd-ha chahn-drah -sah-nah):* Half Moon Pose

Ardha Matsyendrasana *(ahrd-ha maht-see-yen-drah -sah-nah):* Half Spinal Twist Pose

Ardha Padmasana *(ahrd-ha pahd-mah -sah-nah):* Half Lotus Posture

Asana: pose; posture

Ashram: spiritual center for practice and study of Yoga

Ashtanga *(ahsh-tahng-gah):* Eight Limbs

Ashtanga Yoga: Eight Limb Path of yogic practice that emphasizes abstinence, observances, postures, breath control, sense withdrawal, concentration, meditation, and contemplation

Baddha *(bahd-dah):* caught; restrained

Baddha Padamasana *(bahd-dah pahd-mah-sah-nah):* Bound Lotus Posture

Bakasana *(bah-kah -sah-nah):* Crane Posture

Balasana *(bah-lah -sah-nah)*: Child's Pose

Bandha: a muscle "lock" or contraction, used to direct energy throughout the body and stabilize Yoga postures

Bhakti Yoga: path of devotion

Bhujangasana *(bhooj-ahng-gah -sah-nah)*: Cobra Posture

Chakorasana *(chuk-rah-vahk–sah-nah)*: Moonbeam Bird Pose

Chatura: four

Chaturanga Dandasana *(chah-tur-ahng-gah dahn-dah-sah-nah)*: Four Limb Staff Pose

Dandasana *(dahn-dah -sah-nah)*: Staff, Rod, or Stick Pose

Dhanurasana *(dah-nu-rah -sah-nah)*: Bow Posture

Drishti: gazing point; point of focus maintained while in a Yoga posture

Garudasana *(gha-ruh-dah -sah-nah)*: Eagle Pose

Gomukha *(gow-mook-hah)*: cow

Gomukhasana *(gow-mook-hah -sah-nah)*: Cow Head Pose

Guru: teacher

Hala: plough

Halasana: Plough Pose

Hanuman *(hah-nu-mah)*: famous leaping monkey general in Hindu legend

Hanumanasana *(hah-nu-mah -sah-nah)*: Leg Split Pose

Hasta: hand

Hatha: positive and negative life forces; sun and moon; active and receptive life forces

Hatha Yoga: the Yoga of health and physical discipline

Indra: god of thunder, lightning, and rain

Jalandhara bandha: chin lock

Janu *(jah-noo)*: knee

Janu Sirsasana *(jah-noo sheer-shah -sah-nah)*: Head Knee Pose

Japas *(jah-pahs)*: "muttering" recitation of a mantra

Jnana *(gyah-nah)*: sacred knowledge

Jnana Mudra *(gyah-nah moo-drah)*: knowledge seal or lock; a hand placement used in many seated poses

Karma: result of daily action

Karna: ear

Kona: angle

Kundalani: divine cosmic energy

Kumbhaka: retention of breath

Kurmasana *(ker-mah -sah-nah)*: Tortoise Pose

Maharsi: great sage

Marichyasana *(mah-ree-chee-yah -sah-nah)*: one of the seated postures in Ashtanga Yoga named after a sage

Matsyasana *(maht-see-yah -sah-nah)*: Fish Posture

Matsyendra: lord of the fish

Matsyendrasana: Lord of the Fish Pose

Mayurasana *(mah-yoor-ah -sah-nah)*: Peacock Posture

Moola Bandha: root lock or muscle contraction at the base of the spine (also spelled mula bandha)

Nadis *(nah-dees)*: energy channels

Navasana *(nah-wa -sah-nah)*: Boat Posture

Pada *(pahd-ah)*: foot

Padangusthasana *(pahd-anhg-goo-stah -sah-nah)*: Jackknife Pose

Padmasana *(pahd-ma -sah-nah)*: Lotus Posture

Parivritta *(pah-ree-vree-tah)*: revolved; turned around

Parivrtta Parsvakonasana *(pah-ree-vree-tah pahr-shvah-koh-nah -sah-nah)*: Revolved Side Angle Pose (*utthita* is extended)

Parivritta Trikonasana: Twisted Extended Triangle Pose

Parsva *(pahr-shvah)*: side; flank

Parsva Bakasana *(pahr-shvah bah-kah -sah-nah)*: Sideways Crane Pose

Parsvottanasana *(pahrsh-vot-tah-nah -sah-nah)*: Expanded (or Extended) Side Angle Pose (to bless each leg)

Paschima *(pash-chee-mah)*: west

Paschimottanasana *(pash-chee-moh-tah-nah-sah-nah)*: Seated Forward Bend Posture (literally "west stretch")

Prana *(prah-nah)*: life-force; energy (Earth, air, fire, water, ether)

Pranayama *(prah-nah-yah-mah)*: the studied practice of controlled breathing to increase vital life-force energy throughout the body during Yoga

Prasarita *(prah-sah-ree-tah)*: spread out; expanded

Props: pillows, blocks, straps, supports, mats, and other objects that can help you more comfortably perform postures while you build flexibility and strength

Puraka: inhalation

Raja Yoga: Sanskrit meaning "mastering the mind"; the royal path; the path of kings

Rajas: the principle of dynamism

Rajasic foods: hot, spicy, stimulating foods

Rechaka: exhalation

Salabhasana *(shuh-lub-ha-sah-nah)*: Locust Posture

Salamba *(sah-lahm-bah)*: supported

Salamba Sirsasana *(sah-lahm-bah sheer-shah- sah-nah)*: Head Support or Headstand Pose

Sarvanga: the whole body

Sarvangasana: Shoulder Stand

Sattva: the principle of lucidity

Sattvic diet: a diet rich in fresh foods — fruits, vegetables, whole grains, nuts, and seeds; the traditional yogi diet

Savasana *(shah-vah -sah-nah)*: Corpse Pose

Setu *(say-too)*: bridge

Setu Bandha *(say-too bahd-dah)*: Bridge Posture

Siddha: a sage; a semi-divine being of great holiness

Siddhasana *(sid-hah-sah-nah)*: Perfect Posture

Simhasana *(sim-ha -sah-nah)*: Lion Posture

Sirsa *(sheer-shah)*: head

Sirsangusthasana *(sheer-shanhg-goo-stah sah-na)*: Deep Lunge Posture

Sukhasana *(suh-kah -sah-nah)*: Easy Posture

Surya Namaskara *(soor-yah nah-mahs-kah-rah)*: Sun Salutes

Tadasana *(tah-dah-sah-nah)*: Standing Mountain Pose

Tolasana *(toh-lah -sah-nah)*: Scale Pose

Trikona: triangle

Uddiyana Bandha: Sanskrit meaning "flying up"; a muscle contraction of the lower abdomen

Ujjayi breathing: Sanskrit meaning "victorious breathing"; a controlled form of nose-only breathing used to help focus the mind and pace the movements during Yoga practice

Upavishta *(oopah-vish-tah)*: Leg Split Sideways Pose

Urdhva Dhanurasana *(oord-hv dah-nu-rah-sah-nah)*: Wheel Pose

Urdhva Mukha Svanasana *(oord-hvah mook-hah)*: Upward Facing Dog Pose

Ustrasana *(oo-strah -sah-nah)*: Camel Pose

Utkatasana *(oot-kah-tah -sah-nah)*: Powerful Chair Posture

Uttanasana *(oo-tah-nah -sah-nah)*: Standing Forward Bend

Uttihita *(oot-hee-tah)*: raised; extended

Utthita Hasta Padangusthasana *(oot-hee-tah hah-stah pahd-anhg-goo-stah-sah-nah)*: Extended Foot Balance Pose

Utthita Parsvakonasana *(oot-hee-tah pahr-shvah koh-nah -sah-nah)*: Extended Side Angle Pose

Uttihita Trikonasana *(oot-hee-tah tree-koh-nah sah-nah)*: Extended Triangle Pose

Vajra *(vahj-rah)*: thunderbolt; adamantine

Vajrasana *(vahj-rah -sah-nah)*: Kneeling Posture; Thunderbolt Pose

Vinyasa *(veen-yah-sah)*: connecting movements used to keep your body moving, your heart and lungs working, and your body heat up as you switch from one asana to the next

Virabhadrasana *(vee-rah bhuh-drah -sah-nah)*: Warrior Pose

Vrksasana *(vrik-shah -sah-nah)*: Tree Posture

Yoga: union; to yoke

Appendix B
Yoga Resources

● ●

*1*n this series of listings, I provide some of my favorite resources for more information regarding many aspects of the practice of Power Yoga.

Books

Beginner

Astanga Yoga Primer by Baba Hari Dass: www.jivamuktiyoga.com. 404 Lafayette St. 3rd fl., New York, NY 10003; phone 212-353-0214 or 800-295-6814, fax 212-995-1313; e-mail JivaMukt@aol.com

Yoga For Dummies by Georg Feuerstein and Larry Payne. ISBN: 07645551175, Hungry Minds, Inc. 1999. Web site: www.dummies.com

Yoga Journal's Yoga Basics by Mara Carrico. ISBN: 0805045716. Henry Holt & Co. 1997. Yoga Journal, 2054 University Avenue, Berkeley, CA 94704; phone 510-841-9200, fax 510-644-310; Web site: www.yogajournal.com

Yoga: The Spirit and Practice of Moving into Stillness by Erich Schiffmann. ISBN: 061207606. Pocket Books. Web site: www.movingintostillness.com

Yoga, the Ultimate Gift by Doug Swenson. A guide to basic soft-form Yoga practice: www.ashtanga.net

Intermediate to advanced

Beyond Power Yoga by Beryl Bender Birch. ISBN: 0684855267. Simon & Schuster 1999. Web Site: www.power-yoga.com

The Complete Guide to Yoga Adjustments and Partner Work by Doug Swenson: www.ashtanga.net

The Dawn of Yoga Power by Doug Swenson: www.ashtanga.net

Power Yoga by Beryl Bender Birch. ISBN: 0020583516. Macmillan Publishing Co. 1994. Web site: www.power-yoga.com

The Practice Manual by David Swenson. ISBN 1891252089. Ashtanga Yoga Productions. Web site: www.ashtanga.net

Yoga Mala by Sri K. Patthabi Jois. ISBN: 0970050100. Patanjali Yoga Productions 2000. Web site: www.jivamuktiyoga.com

Clothing, Props, Supplies, and Accessories

Barefoot Yoga Supplies (cotton rugs for Power Yoga practice) and Bheka Yoga Supplies (complete line of mats and supplies). 258 A Street, Unit 6B, Ashland, OR 97520; phone 800-366-4541; e-mail bheka@internetcds.com, Web sites: www.bheka.com or www.barefootyoga.com

Blue Canoe (makers of organic cotton clothing perfect for Yoga practice). P.O. Box 543, Garberville, CA 95542-0543; phone 888-923-1373, 707-923-1373; Web site www.bluecanoe.com

Hugger Mugger Yoga Products (complete line of products and clothing). 3937 S. Five Hundred W. Salt Lake City, Utah 84123; Inside the U.S. 800-473-4888, Outside the U.S. 801-268-9642, Fax 801-268-2629; e-mail comments@huggermugger.com, Web site www.huggermugger.com

Prana (clothing for Yoga and climbing). 2077 Las Palmas Dr., Carlsbad, CA 92009; Phone 800-557-7262 or 760-431-8015; e-mail info@prana.com; Web site www.prana.com

Yoga Zone (Yoga supplies and clothing). e-mail info@yogazone.com, Web site www.yogazone.com

Magazines

Ascent Magazine: Box 9, Kootenay Bay, British Columbia, CANADA, V0B 1X0; phone 800-661-8711 or 250-227-9224, Fax 250-227-9494; US subscription office, P.O. Box 160. Porthill, ID 85853 U.S.A.; e-mail info@ascentmagazine.com, Web site www.ascentmagazine.com

Natural Health: USA: 1 year (9 issues) for $17.95, Outside of the US: 1 year (9 issues) for $29.95 U.S.; Web site www.naturalhealthmag.com

New Age: New Age Publishing, 42 Pleasant St, Watertown, MA 02472; phone 800-782-7006 or 617-926-0200, fax 617-926-5021; e-mail editor@newage.com, Web site www.newage.com

Yoga Connoisseur (online magazine): Yoga Connoisseur Magazine, 368 Avery St., Ashland, OR 97520; e-mail info@yogacritic.com, Web site www.yogacritic.com

Yoga International: One Year $18.00; Yoga International, RR 1 Box 407, Honesdale, PA 18431; phone 800-253-6243 ext. 3, Fax 570-253-6360; e-mail info@yimag.org, Web site www.yimag.org

Yoga Journal: One year (seven issues) $14.95; Yoga Journal, P.O. Box 469088, Escondido, CA 92046-9088; To call subscription customer service 800-600-YOGA, (8:30 a.m. - 5:00 p.m. PST) or 760-796-6549; Web site www.yogajournal.com

Yoga Online (online magazine): Web site indigo.ie/~cmouze/yoga_online/yoga_online.htm

Retreat Centers and Ashrams

Ashtanga Yoga Center, Tim Miller, Director, Retreats in Hawaii, Mexico, and Bali. 118 West E Street, Encinitas, CA 92024; phone 760-632-7093; e-mail ashtangayoga@home.com, Web site www.ashtangayogacenter.com

Ashtanga Yoga Productions. David and Doug Swenson Each of us offer Power Yoga workshops throughout the U.S. and in exotic locations throughout the world. P.O. Box 680404, Houston, TX 77268; phone 800-684-6927 or 510-632-2007; e-mail info@ashtanga.net, or dougtahoe@hotmail.com, Web site www.ashtanga.net

Feathered Pipe Foundation, P.O. Box 1682, Helena, MT 59624; phone 406-442-8196, Fax 406-442-8110; e-mail fpranch@mt.net, Web site www.featheredpipe.com

The Hard and the Soft Astanga Yoga Institute, Beryl Bender Birch and Tom Birch, Power Yoga retreats in New York City and East Hampton, NY and Jamaica. P.O. Box 5009, East Hampton, NY 11937. e-mail: yoga@power-yoga.com, Web site www.power-yoga.com

Hippocrates Health Institute, Institute, 1443 Palmdale Court, West Palm Beach, FL 33411; phone 561-471-8876, reservations only 800-842-2125, fax 561-471-9464; Web site www.hippocratesinst.com

Institute Learning Center, Ann Wigmore Mailing address: PO Box 429, Rincón, Puerto Rico 00677, Physical address: Carretera 115, Km. 20, Calle Moret, Bo. Guayabo, Aguada, Puerto Rico 00602; phone 787-868-6307 or 868-0591, Fax 787-868-2430; e-mail wigmore@coqui.net, Web site www.annwigmore.org

Mount Madonna Center, 445 Summit Rd, Watsonville, CA 95076; phone 408-847-0406, Fax 408-847-2683; e-mail programs@mountmadonna.org, Web site www.mountmadonna.org

Danny Paradise Yoga workshops around the world; contact: Ian Macdonald, 70 Southmoor Road, Oxford, England 0X2 6RB; e-mail macdonaldreynell@netscapeonline.co.uk; Diane Bruni and Marshal Linfoot: e-mail info@downwarddog.com

Poweryoga.com, Bryan Kest, Retreats in the U.S. and Peru. 1247 Lincoln Blvd., #241, Santa Monica, CA 90401-1711; phone 310-458-0830, fax 310-282-8295; e-mail info@poweryoga.com, Web site www.poweryoga.com

Shoshoni Yoga Retreat, P.O. Box 410, Rollinsville, CO 80474; phone 303-642-0116; e-mail kailasa@shoshoni.org, Web site www.shoshoni.org

Sivananda Ashtam Centers: Sivananda Yoga Vedanta Center, 243 West Twenty Fourth Street, New York, NY 10011, and worldwide; phone 212-255-4560, Fax 212-727-7392; e-mail NewYork@sivananda.org, Web site www.sivananda.org

Tree of Life Rejuvenation Center, P.O. Box 1080, Patagonia, AZ 85624; phone 520-394-2520 or 520-394-0067, Fax 520-394-2099; e-mail Healing@Treeoflife.nu, Web site www.treeoflife.nu

The Yoga Workshop, Richard Freeman Ashtanga retreats in Colorado, Hawaii, Utah, Bali, and other locations. 2020 Twenty First St., Boulder, Colorado 80302; phone 303-449-6102; e-mail Yogaworkshop@mindspring.com, Web site www.yogaworkshop.com

Tapes

Audio

Ashtanga Yoga Productions, P.O. Box 680404, Houston, TX 77268; phone 800-684-6927 or 510-632-2007; e-mail info@ashtanga.net, Web site www.ashtanga.net

The Dawn of Yoga Power by Doug Swenson. A good beginner-level Power Yoga routine with a deep relaxation.

Just Relax by David Swenson. Relaxing Yoga for all levels.

Poetic Flow Power Ashtanga by Doug Swenson. Intermediate; audio of my unique poetic flow of first-level Power Ashtanga.

Soothing Touch of Power Level II by Doug Swenson. Advanced; a challenging audiotape that presents Power Yoga in a soft-form format.

Teacher Training Lecture/Question and Answer by Doug Swenson. Teacher training; informative and educational advice for all those who teach Yoga.

Yoga: The Practice, First Series by David Swenson. Intermediate; the entire primary series of Ashtanga Yoga.

Yoga: The Practice, Second and Third Series by David Swenson. Advanced; a challenging intermediate series of Ashtanga Yoga workouts, focusing on backbends, inversions, and hip openers.

Yoga: Short Forms by David Swenson. Abbreviated versions of the Ashtanga Primary Series for beginners or people with tight schedules.

Baptiste Power Yoga Institute, 2000 Massachusetts Ave. Cambridge, MA 02140; phone 617-441-2144; e-mail product@baronbaptiste.com

Teacher Training Series 1 by Baron Baptiste. Teacher training; advice on how to successfully share the experience of Power Yoga.

Video

Ashtanga Yoga Productions, P.O. Box 680404, Houston, TX 77268; phone 800-684-6927 or 510-632-2007; e-mail info@ashtanga.net, Web site www.ashtanga.net

Dawn of Yoga Power by Doug Swenson. Power Yoga for the beginner.

Just Relax by David Swenson. Relaxing Yoga for all levels, but great for beginners.

Poetic Flow Power Ashtanga by Doug Swenson. A representation of my unique and flowing approach to Power Ashtanga for beginners to strong intermediates.

A Practical Guide to the Path of Yoga, Health and Fitness by Doug Swenson. A great video for those who strive for total body health, with Yoga as a base.

The Soothing Touch of Power by Doug Swenson. A combination of Powerful Yoga with a soft-form format that offers a challenging but soothing Yoga workout.

Yoga: The Practice, First Series by David Swenson. The entire primary series of Ashtanga Yoga.

Yoga The Practice Second and Third Series by David Swenson. The very challenging intermediate series of Ashtanga Yoga, where the focus changes to backbends, inversions, and hip openers.

Yoga: Short Forms by David Swenson. Abbreviated versions of the Ashtanga Primary Series for beginners or people with tight schedules.

Baptiste Power Yoga Institute, 2000 Massachusetts Ave., Cambridge, MA 02140; phone 617-441-2144; e-mail product@baronbaptiste.com.

Power Yoga for Beginners by Baron Baptiste. A challenging introduction to Power Yoga.

Power Yoga, the Next Challenge by Baron Baptiste. The third video in Baron Baptiste's line of videos; a modified version of Ashtanga Yoga.

Power Yoga, the Ultimate Yoga Workout by Baron Baptiste. The second video in Baron Baptiste's line of videos; more challenging than the first.

Moving Into Stillness, 2407 18th Street, Santa Monica, CA 90405; phone 310-399-8803; e-mail: erichyog@earthlink.net; Web site: www.movingintostillness.com

Ali MacGraw Yoga Mind and Body with Erich Schiffmann. A beautiful workout.

Moving Into Stillness by Erich Schiffmann.

Poweryoga.com, 1247 Lincoln Blvd., #241, Santa Monica, CA 90401-1711; phone 310-458-0830, fax 310-282-8295; e-mail info@poweryoga.com, Web site www.poweryoga.com

Power Yoga Volume 1 by Bryan Kest. The first in Bryan's series of challenging Power Yoga workouts; designed to energize.

Power Yoga Volume 2 by Bryan Kest. The second in Bryan's series of videos; designed to tone.

Power Yoga Volume 3 by Bryan Kest. The most challenging of Bryan Kest's videotapes; designed to make you sweat.

The Yoga Workshop, 2020 Twenty First St., Boulder, Colorado 80302, USA; phone 303-449-6102; e-mail Yogaworkshop@mindspring.com, Web site www.yogaworkshop.com

Yoga Breathing and Relaxation by Richard Freeman. A detailed introduction to the Ashtanga Primary Series.

Yoga with Richard Freeman: Ashtanga Yoga, The Primary Series by Richard Freeman. The entire primary series of Ashtanga Yoga.

Web Sites

www.ashtanga.com: Ashtanga Yoga news and events, and a list of Ashtanga studios

www.ashtanga.net: David Swenson's Ashtanga site with a calendar of David's and my workshops, retreats, books, videos, and audios

www.omplace.com: A complete alternative directory, and publishers of an e-mail newsletter for health and wellness

www.power-yoga.com: Beryl Bender Birch's site about Power Yoga, listing her books and schedule

www.poweryoga.com: Bryan Kest's Power Yoga site, which includes lists of his videotapes and schedule

www.yogadirectory.com: A searchable directory of Yoga resources for all aspects of physical and spiritual Yoga, including studios, books, and supplies

www.yogafinder.com: A searchable directory of Yoga studios around the globe

www.yogaworkshop.com: Richard Freeman's Ashtanga Yoga site

Index

Y

Notes

Notes

Notes

Notes

Notes

Notes

Notes

Notes